AF183097

FOCUS ON PARKINSON'S DISEASE RESEARCH

Focus on Parkinson's Disease Research

Marianne J. Willow
Editor

Nova Science Publishers, Inc.
New York

Copyright © 2006 by Nova Science Publishers, Inc.

All rights reserved. No part of this book may be reproduced, stored in a retrieval system or transmitted in any form or by any means: electronic, electrostatic, magnetic, tape, mechanical photocopying, recording or otherwise without the written permission of the Publisher.

For permission to use material from this book please contact us:
Telephone 631-231-7269; Fax 631-231-8175
Web Site: http://www.novapublishers.com

NOTICE TO THE READER

The Publisher has taken reasonable care in the preparation of this book, but makes no expressed or implied warranty of any kind and assumes no responsibility for any errors or omissions. No liability is assumed for incidental or consequential damages in connection with or arising out of information contained in this book. The Publisher shall not be liable for any special, consequential, or exemplary damages resulting, in whole or in part, from the readers' use of, or reliance upon, this material.

This publication is designed to provide accurate and authoritative information with regard to the subject matter covered herein. It is sold with the clear understanding that the Publisher is not engaged in rendering legal or any other professional services. If legal or any other expert assistance is required, the services of a competent person should be sought. FROM A DECLARATION OF PARTICIPANTS JOINTLY ADOPTED BY A COMMITTEE OF THE AMERICAN BAR ASSOCIATION AND A COMMITTEE OF PUBLISHERS.

LIBRARY OF CONGRESS CATALOGING-IN-PUBLICATION DATA

Focus on Parkinson's disease research / Marianne J. Willow, editor.
p. ; cm.
Includes bibliographical references and index.
ISBN 1-59454-924-9
1. Parkinson's disease--Research. 2. Brain--Diseases--Research.
I. Willow, Marianne J.
[DNLM: 1. Parkinson Disease. WL 359 F652 2006]
RC382.F63 2006
616.8'330072--dc22 2005037227

Published by Nova Science Publishers, Inc. ✣ New York

CONTENTS

PREFACE

Parkinson's disease (PD) is characterized by an insidious onset with slowing of emotional and voluntary movement, muscular rigidity, postural abnormality and tremor. Parkinson's disease was first described in 1817 by James Parkinson. It is a progressive, neurological disease mainly affecting people over the age of 50, although at least 10% of cases occur at an earlier age. It affects people of either sex and all ethnic groups. In the normal brain, some nerve cells produce the chemical dopamine, which transmits signals within the brain to produce smooth movement of muscles. In Parkinson's patients, 80% or more of these dopamine-producing cells are damaged, dead, or otherwise degenerated. This causes the nerve cells to fire wildly, leaving patients unable to control their movements. This new book brings together the latest research in this field.

Despite the recent advances in the discovery of α synuclein gene and parkin gene which help to elucidate the pathogenesis of hereditary Parkinson's disease in some families, the aetiology of Parkinson's disease remains unclear in the majority of the sporadic onset cases. Both environmental and genetic risk factors are thought to be involved and these factors are thought to interact in causing Parkinson's disease. Chapter I reviews and compares the evidence in literature of the cytochrome P450 2D6 (CYP2D6 debrisoquine 4-hydroxylase) genetic polymorphism in Caucasian and Asian populations and the association with Parkinson's disease.

As discussed in Chapter II, Parkinson's disease (PD) is a common progressive neurological disorder that is characterized pathologically by the degeneration of dopaminergic neurons in the substantia nigra pars compacta (SNpc) and elsewhere. It is known that dopamine neurotransmitter is chemically reactive and its oxidation products are highly neurotoxic. It is believed that the novel mechanistic understandings developed here may also offer insights into the pathogenic mechanisms of other age-dependent neurodegenerative diseases.

Parkinson's disease (PD) is a neurodegenerative condition, characterized by motor deficits such as rigidity, tremor, bradykinesia and geit difficulties as well as non-motor symptoms such as cognitive, mood and behavior changes. Recently it has been shown that testosterone may improve refractory non-motor symptoms of PD. Chapter III will review the current evidence that estrogen and testosterone may play a role in neurodegenerative diseases such as PD.

To elucidate the change in neuronal function with movement dysfunction occurring after the administration of a dopamine antagonist, the potency of high-resolution single photon emission computed tomography (SPECT) was estimated using an animal model in which Parkinsonian symptoms gradually progressed following chronic treatment with the antipsychotic haloperidol (HP). These results suggested that, using noninvasive imaging techniques, dopaminergic neuronal change could be detected in Parkinsonian syndrome induced by long-term treatment with D_2R-binding antipsychotics. These results are reported in Chapter IV.

Chapter V discusses how Parkinson's disease is a progressive neurodegenerative disease involving loss of dopaminergic neurons in the substantia nigra of the midbrain. Dopaminergic neurons appear to die by a process of necrosis or apoptosis that is induced by oxidative stress. There is, however, a theoretical basis for the use of aldehyde dehydrogenase inhibitors to slow down the progression of the disease. Future treatment of Parkinson's disease could consider the inhibition of oxygen radical formation in dopaminergic neurons or ways to stimulate DNA repair and prevent cell death.

As reported in Chapter VI, there is a group of neurological disorders that pulmonary principles can be applied. In this group, pulmonary dysfunction often complicates a variety of musculoskeletal, medical and central nervous system disorders, including travmatic brain injury, stroke, multiple sclerosis and Parkinson's Disease (PD). Patients with PD with a variety of symptoms such as dyspnea on exertion, decreased exercise tolerance, difficulties during activities of daily living, mood changes, hypoxemia have been shown to benefit from pulmonary rehabilitation program.

In: Focus on Parkinson's Disease Research
Editor: Marianne J. Willow, pp. 1-19
ISBN 1-59454-924-9
© 2006 Nova Science Publishers, Inc.

Chapter I

REVIEW, COMPARISON AND META-ANALYSIS OF CYP2D6 POLYMORPHISM AND ASSOCATION WITH PARKINSON'S DISEASE IN CAUCASIAN AND ASIAN POPULATIONS

Daniel Kam Yin Chan[1,*], Dennis Cordato[2] and Wai Tak Hung[3]
[1]Department of Aged Care & Rehabilitation, Bankstown-Lidcombe Hospital
(University of New South Wales & University of Western Sydney), Sydney, Australia
[2]Department of Neurology, Bankstown-Lidcombe Hospital, Sydney, Australia
[3]Key University Research Strength in Health Technologies, University of Technology, Broadway, Sydney, Australia

ABSTRACT

Despite the recent advances in the discovery of α synuclein gene and parkin gene which help to elucidate the pathogenesis of hereditary Parkinson's disease in some families, the aetiology of Parkinson's disease remains unclear in the majority of the sporadic onset cases. Both environmental and genetic risk factors are thought to be involved and these factors are thought to interact in causing Parkinson's disease. The hypothesis that failure to metabolise xenobiotics is a putative risk factor in predisposed individuals with susceptible genetic defects remain an attractive possibility. This hypothesis is further supported by some drug addicts who developed parkinsonism after self-administrating synthetic meperidine analogues contaminated with 1-methyl-4-phenyl-1,2,3,6-tetrahydropyridine. This paper reviews and compares the evidence in literature of the cytochrome P450 2D6 (CYP2D6 debrisoquine 4-hydroxylase) genetic polymorphism in Caucasian and Asian populations and the association with Parkinson's disease. Furthermore, it also attempts to clarify the issue by using meta-analyses for analysing the

* Correspondence concerning this article should be addressed to Prof. Daniel Kam Yin Chan, Department of Aged Care & rehabilitation Bankstown Lidcombe Hospital (University of New South Wales & University of Western Sydney) Bankstown, NSW 2200 Australia.

results of genotypic studies of CYP2D6 and Parkinson's disease in the two populations. Interestingly, this latest and largest meta-analysis showed that there is a weak association of CYP2D6 poor metaboliser genotype and Parkinson's disease in Caucasians (Odds ratio 1.3; 95% CI: 1.04 – 1.63). However, the situation is less clear in Asians as the poor metaboliser genotype is very rare and meta-analysis of heterozygotes in Asians carrying one mutant gene (instead of two) indicated an increased risk of 2.07 (95% CI 1.33 - 3.24) compared to controls. However, the results of poor metaboliser genotypes in Caucasians and heterozygotes in Asians are clouded by the fact that there is significant heterogeneity amongst the studies used in the meta-analyses. Therefore, although the meta-analysis did overcome the sample size problems of allele association studies, other limitations remain including the lack of consideration of environmental factors, lack of consideration of interactions, diagnostic accuracy for Parkinson's disease and consideration of multiple genes being involved.

Keywords: CYP2D6 polymorphism, meta-analysis, Parkinson's disease

Introduction

The aetiology of Parkinson's disease remains unclear in the majority of cases. With the exception of about 5% of cases that have a definite genetic inheritance pattern, and 10-15%, which have a familial clustering, the vast majority of Parkinson's disease cases are of sporadic in onset. A 'purely' environmental explanation for sporadic onset Parkinson's disease is also lacking. However, 'toxic' parkinsonism is well established as seen in cases of neuroleptic-induced parkinsonism, carbon monoxide or manganese intoxication, and anoxia to the globus pallidus or substantia nigra. Environmental factors in the general population such as herbicide/pesticide exposure have also been reported to increase the risk of Parkinson's disease whereas other environmental factors, most notably cigarette smoking, have been reported to be potential 'protective' factors [1]. The discovery of 1-methyl-4-phenyl-1,2,3,6-tetrahydropyridine (MPTP) induced parkinsonism in intravenous drug users [2] further supports the concept that potential putative environmental factors exist and also that gene-environment interactions are probably important in the aetiology of Parkinson's disease.

MPTP was first recognized as a cause of parkinsonism in 1976 after a chemistry student presented with catatonia, mutism and rigidity following self-administration of synthetic meperidine analogues contaminated with MPTP [3]. MPTP induces a form of parkinsonism which is clinically indistinguishable from the common forms of Parkinson's disease although pathologically its lacks the hallmark presence of Lewy bodies [4]. However not all subjects who have been exposed to MPTP develop parkinsonism. Indeed only a small proportion of exposed individuals have acquired the disease. This raised the possibility of different genetic susceptibility amongst individuals.

The search for putative environmental factors has resulted in the recognition that genetic polymorphisms of enzymes and/or proteins involved in the metabolism or transport of dopamine as well as detoxifying enzymes involved in drug and xenobiotic metabolism may be associated with an increased risk of Parkinson's disease. For example, monoamine oxidase

B (MAO-B) has been extensively studied by virtue of its role in the metabolism of dopamine and conversion of MPTP to the active neurotoxic metabolite 1-methyl-4-phenylpyridinium ion (MPP^+) [5]. Other susceptibility gene polymorphisms that may involve drug and xenobiotic metabolism and have been associated with Parkinson's disease include N-acetyltransferase 2 and glutathione s-transferase M1 [6]. However, studies of genetic susceptibility to sporadic Parkinson's disease for a large number of these susceptibility genes have yielded contradictory results. One of the most widely studied susceptibility genes is cytochrome P450 mono-oxygenase (CYP2D6). The 4-hydroxylation of the antihypertensive debrisoquine by CYP2D6 was the first genetic polymorphism in the metabolism of a drug to be reported in association with the cytochrome P450 enzyme system in humans [7]. This gene is located on chromosome 22q13 (ch22q13). Several polymorphisms of this gene have resulted in similar gene expression with poor metabolism of debrisoquine 4-hydroxylase [8-10]. Variant alleles CYP2D6*4 (B allele in old nomenclature) and CYP2D*3 (A allele in old nomenclature) comprise approximately 90% of the individuals with low debrisoquine 4-hydroxylase activity [9,10]. CYP2D6 substrates are structurally diverse; most are small molecules that interact with the enzyme via electrostatic forces between a basic nitrogen atom, which is common to the majority of CYP2D6 substrates, including neurotoxicant MPTP, and an aspartic acid residue in the active site of the enzyme [11].

CYP2D6 metabolises many xenobiotics including the β-blocking agents (propranolol, metoprolol), antiarrhythmics (flecainide, mexiletine), tricyclic antidepressants (imipramine, nortriptyline) and other miscellaneous drugs such as the antipsychotic haloperidol, the analgesic agent codeine and the neurotoxin MPTP [12,13]. In vitro studies have shown that MPTP and MPP^+ bind to and are metabolised by CYP2D6 [14], which is localised to substantia nigra of the brain [15]. The activity of CYP2D6 is genetically determined and two distinct subgroups are recognised. The term poor metaboliser is used to describe those people who have impaired or undetectable CYP2D6 activity. This phenotype is inherited as autosomal recessive trait. Although there are more than 40 alleles reported so far, over 95% of the poor metaboliser phenotypes in Caucasians are secondary to the following three polymorphisms [10] (in order of frequency): G to A (G1934A) transition at the intron 3/exon 4 junction (CYP2D6*4, old nomenclature CYP2D6B), which results in a mRNA maturation defect [10], base pair (A2637) deletion in exon 5 (CYP2D6*3, old nomenclature CYP2D6A) and, rarely, deletion of the entire gene (CYP2D6*5, old nomenclature CYP2D6D) [16]. Individuals with any two defective alleles are classified as having the poor metaboliser genotype.

It is estimated that about 5 to 10% of Caucasian populations are of poor metaboliser phenotypes [17]. Therefore, the CYP2D6 mutant allele is certainly not uncommon and if indeed the poor metaboliser phenotype predisposes individuals to Parkinson's disease, then the impact on the population as a whole cannot be underestimated. In contrast, the frequency of a poor metaboliser phenotype amongst Asian populations is much lower at approximately 1% (or less) suggesting that this putative gene may be less important in the aetiology of Parkinson's disease amongst Asians or alternatively, its low frequency may partly explain a lower prevalence of Parkinson's disease in Asians [18].

History

Barbeau et al [19] first suggested that poor metaboliser phenotypes may have an increased susceptibility to Parkinson's disease because of impaired detoxification of neurotoxins. This hypothesis was supported initially by pharmacokinetic studies of CYP2D6 activity [19]. However, the results were flawed by the confounding influence on CYP2D6 activity of antiparkinsonian drug therapy, and not supported by subsequent studies [20,21]. Furthermore, there were other limitations of pharmacokinetic assays such as the accuracy of biochemical measurements, which can affect the determination of extensive or poor metaboliser status. Investigations using DNA-based genetic assays can overcome such confounding effects. Therefore, since the 1990's, the ascertainment of metaboliser status of CYP2D6 by pharmacokinetic assays, have largely been replaced by genotypic studies. Although genotypic studies can overcome some of the shortcomings of phenotypic studies of CYP2D6 activities, the results of genotypic studies have similarly been inconsistent because other limitations remain. Some of these studies have limited statistical power and have used different techniques (restriction fragment length polymorphism analysis vs polymerase chain reaction based DNA amplification) and diagnostic criteria. Thus, the association of the poor metaboliser genotype with Parkinson's disease remains an important but unresolved issue.

Review of Previous Meta-Analysis Studies of CYP2D6 Association with Parkinson's Disease in Caucasians and Asians

Four meta-analyses studies have been identified using MEDLINE and EMBASE. The first of such meta-analysis was from McCann et al [22]. This report only looked at Caucasian populations. Thirteen reports were found in this meta-analysis. The studies of Tsuneoka et al [23] along with Kondo and Kanazawa [24] were excluded because they examined Asian populations, in whom the poor metaboliser genotype is extremely rare. The study of Akhmedova et al [25] was also excluded from the McCann et al meta-analysis study because only one poor metaboliser genotype was found in the entire population cohort of 150. A net total of ten studies were in the final analysis and all were genotypic studies. The results of the meta-analysis were:

* Total Parkinson's disease patients = 1,133
* Total controls = 1,950
* The odds ratio for the poor metaboliser genotype was 1.47 (95% CI: 1.18-1.96, p = 0.01)
* The odds ratio for the CYP2D6*4 allele was 1.14 (95% CI: 0.98-1.30, p = 0.06)

The odds ratio would have been lower if the study of Akhmedova et al was also included.

The second meta-analysis study was from Rostami-Hodjegan et al [26]. MEDLINE and BIDS EMBASE were used in this study. Both genotypic and phenotypic studies were included. Thirty-five reports on CYP2D6 were found. Eighteen studies of Caucasian subjects were included in the final analyses, of which 11 were genotypic and 7 were phenotypic studies. The remaining reports on CYP2D6 were excluded because of repeated publication, no controls, lack of specific data on number of poor metabolisers and studies on Asian subjects. The results of the meta-analysis were:

* Total Parkinson's disease patients and controls = 5,121 (no detail was provided as to the breakdown in numbers of Parkinson's disease subjects and controls)
* The odds ratio for poor metabolisers (genotype and phenotype combined) was 1.32 (95% CI: 0.98-1.78), which was of borderline statistical significance because the confidence interval crossed unity.

The third meta-analysis study was by Christensen et al [27]. Case-control and cohort studies were identified in searches on MEDLINE, EMBASE, Toxline and Reference Update. Twenty-one studies (both phenotypic and genotypic) were identified of which six were excluded because they were not reported as full papers (n = 3), used incomplete genotype analysis (n = 2) or used Parkinson's disease patients as both control individuals and cases (n = 1). Fifteen studies (8 phenotypic, 7 genotypic), which included one phenotypic study on Chinese subjects, were grouped together in the final analysis. The results of the meta-analysis were as follows:

* Total Parkinson's disease patients = 1,196
* Total controls = 2,364
* The overall odds ratio for the poor metabolisers (phenotype and genotype combined) was 1.48 (95% CI 1.1-1.99).

The fourth meta-analysis was amongst Asians only [28]. A Medline search was conducted and only articles published in English and studies performed in Asian populations were chosen. Eleven articles were identified; two were excluded from analysis, one article was excluded due to lack of availability in English and the other article due to duplication. Their final analysis included 9 articles. The polymorphism of CYP2D6*4 was extremely rare and many studies combined heterozygotes and homozygotes in the calculation of odds ratio. This is a problem in that heterozygotes, unlike homozygotes, are not poor metabolisers and hence should not be grouped but considered separately. The results of the meta-analysis were:

* Total Parkinson's disease patients = 880
* Total controls = 1,864
* The directionality of the odds ratios generated varied from a protective estimate of 0.56 to a risk factor of 2.15 upon comparison of Parkinson's disease cases with controls. The overall odds ratio for the pooled sample was 0.84 (95% CI 0.66 – 1.08). The authors concluded that there was no evidence to support an association of CYP2D6 polymorphism and Parkinson's disease in Asians.

New Meta-Analysis Studies of the Association of CYP2D6 with Parkinson's Disease in Caucasians and Asians

Two of the first three meta-analyses above found that there may be a weak association of the poor metaboliser of CYP2D6 and Parkinson's disease. However, the odds ratio was probably at best = 1.48 (Christensen et al [27]). Two of the meta-analyses also included phenotypic studies, which made comparison with the third one (genotypic study only) difficult. In addition, since the publication of the last meta-analysis report in 1998, there have been a number of additional studies including one sizable study of 576 Parkinson's disease patients (Payami et al [29]). It is therefore timely to review the latest literature and to make an effort to clarify the issue further. Hence, we have attempted a new cumulative meta-analysis study by also including papers that had been published after the three meta-analyses.

We report the latest and largest meta-analysis study of the association of the poor metaboliser genotype of CYP2D6 with Parkinson's disease to date, firstly by analyzing the Caucasian results and secondly by analyzing the Asian results.

Methods

A MEDLINE and EMBASE search from 1983-2003 was performed to find any article reporting the association between the poor metaboliser genotype and Parkinson's disease. Key words used were Parkinson's' disease, CYP2D6, debrisoquine 4-hydroxylase, and genetics. Criteria for inclusion in the analysis were: case-control studies, accepted methods of diagnosing Parkinson's disease studies of Caucasian or Asian subjects and publication in English. Exclusion criteria were non-Caucasian and non-Asian subjects, phenotypic studies of CYP2D6 or not published in English. The Mantel-Haenzsel test was used to estimate the odds ratio in the meta-analysis.

In addition, we had also extracted data from previous meta-analyses, which included publications prior to 1998. We reported and analysed the Caucasian and Asian results. Hence, this study represents the latest and largest meta-analysis study of the association of the poor metaboliser CYP2D6 genotype with Parkinson's disease. We separated the Caucasian results from the Asians' because of differences in prevalence of poor metaboliser genotypes and differences in previous meta-analyses results.

The data were analyzed with the R statistical software [30]. The rmeta package contributed by Thomas Lumley has the function called meta.MH for analysing fixed effects (Mantel-Haenszel) meta-analysis. It was used to compute the individual odds ratio and its 95% C.I. Also, the Mantel-Haenszel summary, and Woolf's test for heterogeneity were computed.

There is still debate concerning what to do with the results of independent studies if when their results are found to be to be significantly heterogenous [31]. Becker and Hedges [32] have admitted: "It is not necessarily inadvisable to draw inference from heterogeneous effects." It is on this basis that we combined heterogeneous studies together for meta-analysis in our study.

Table 1. New meta-analysis of studies investigating the association of CYP2D6 poor metaboliser genotypic polymorphisms with Parkinson's disease in Caucasians.

Study	Poor metaboliser (no. of patients)	Odds ratio for poor metaboliser (95% CI)	CYP2D6*4 and/or CYP2D6*3 number of alleles (results are for 2D6*4 only unless specified)	Odds ratio (95% CI)
Agundez et al (1995) [38]				
Patients (P) = 123	2	0.48	32/246	1.13
Controls (C) = 150	5	(0.09-2.51)	35/300	(0.68-1.89)
Armstrong et al (1992) [54]				
P = 53	2	1.37	23/106	2.38
C = 72	2	(0.19-10.07)	15/144	(1.18-4.83)
Atkinson et al (1999) [53]				
P = 33	2	1.52	18/66	2.44
C = 75	3	(0.25-9.73)	20/150	(1.19-5.00)
Bon et al (1999) * [44]				
P=50	N/A	N/A	41/100	2.34
C=96			44/192	(1.39-3.94)
Bordet et al (1996) [55]				
P = 105	5	1.26	34/210	0.85
C = 105	4	(0.33-4.84)	39/210	(0.51-1.40)
Diederich et al (1996) [56]				
P = 80	3	0.55	31/160	0.97
C = 106	7	(0.14-2.20)	42/212	(0.58-1.63)
Gasser et al (1996) [57]				
P = 178	10	1.39	70/356	0.99
C = 73	3	(0.37-5.20)	29/146	(0.61-1.60)
Harhangi et al (2001) † [58]				
P = 80	8	1.46	31/160	0.73
C = 156	11	(0.56-3.80)	77/312	(0.46-1.17)
Joost et al (1999) * [40]				
P = 109	4	1.01	55/218	1.24
C = 110	4	(0.25-4.14)	47/220	(0.80-1.94)
Kurth and Kurth (1995) [59]				
P = 50	5	1.93	33/100	1.86
C = 110	6	(0.56-6.64)	46/220	(1.10-3.16)
Lucotte et al (1996) [60]				
P = 47	5	5.48	23/94	2.72
C = 47	1	(0.61-48.80)	10/94	(1.21-6.10)
Maraganore et al (2000) [61]				
P = 139	9	1.50	53/274	0.90
C = 113	5	(0.49-4.60)	47/224	(0.58-1.39)
McCann et al (1997) [22]				
P = 112	14	1.70	47/224	1.17
C = 206	16	(0.80-3.62)	76/412	(0.78-1.76)
Nicholl et al (1999) [62]				
P=176	15	0.99	53/352	1.17
C=175	15	(0.47-2.10)	46/350	(0.77-1.79)
Payami et al (2001) [29]				
P = 576	29	0.77	231/1152	0.95
C = 247	16	(0.41-1.44)	103/494	(0.73-1.24)

Table 1. Continued

Study	Poor metaboliser (no. of patients)	Odds ratio for poor metaboliser (95% CI)	CYP2D6*4 and/or CYP2D6*3 number of alleles (results are for 2D6*4 only unless specified)	Odds ratio (95% CI)
Plante-Bordeneuve et al (1994) [63]				
P = 48	5	1.35	24/96	1.50
C = 88	7	(0.40-4.49)	32/176	(0.82-2.73)
Sandy et al (1996) [64]				
P = 108	6	0.76	31/216	0.69
C = 236	17	(0.29-1.98)	92/472	(0.44-1.08)
Sabbagh et al (1999) † [39]				
P = 109	6	0.82	33/218	0.85
C = 514	34	(0.34-2.01)	179/1028	(0.56-1.27)
Smith et al (1992) [65]				
P = 229	27	2.54	103/458	1.23
C = 720	36	(1.51-4.28)	275/1440	(0.95-1.59)
Stefanovic et al (2000) † [42]				
P = 41	3	5.64	18/82	1.98
C = 145	2	(0.91-35.00)	36/290	(1.06-3.72)
Wilhelmsen et al (1997) [46]				
P = 121	6	1.39	45/242	1.09
C = 138	5	(0.41-4.67)	48/276	(0.69-1.70)

Bold characters represent new studies not previously included in meta-analysis published.
† refers to combined CYP2D6*3 and CYP2D6*4 results.

Results

Twenty-one reports (for references see Table 1) were found to be eligible for inclusion in the final analysis of the Caucasian arm of the study, and of these ten were not analysed in any of the previous meta-analysis studies. Asian studies were considered separately because of the rarity of the poor metaboliser genotype. Likewise, the study of Akhmedova et al [25] was excluded because only one poor metaboliser genotype was found in the entire study population of 150.

The new meta-analysis study for Caucasians consisted of 2567 patients with Parkinson's disease and 3682 subjects who were controls. Analysis of this new study showed that there was still a statistically significant result for Caucasians who are poor metaboliser in genotype and an association with Parkinson's disease. The Mantel-Haenszel odds ratio was 1.3 (95% CI: 1.04 – 1.63) but Woolf's test for heterogeneity was heterogeneous = 19.9 (p value = 0.3998), therefore indicating that there is some doubt as to the validity of the meta-analysis result. As for CYP2D6*4 allele frequency, the result was less convincing as the value of Mantel-Haenszel odds ratio just exceeded unity = 1.13 (95% CI: 1.03 – 1.25). The Woolf's test for heterogeneity = 43.28 (p value = 0.0019, therefore homogeneous). Further details of the study can be found in Table 1.

For the Asian arm of the meta-analysis eleven articles were identified (for references see table 2); one article [33] was excluded due to non-English publication, two articles [34,35] were excluded because of duplications, and two others were excluded because the mutations examined were rare [36,37]. The net results of the remaining six Asian studies were analysed. The total number of Parkinson's disease was 568 and the total for controls was 876. Using Mantel-Haenszel χ^2 test, the odds ratio for possessing one mutant allele of either CYP2D6*4 or CYP2D6*10 in Asians is associated with an increased risk of 2.07 (95% CI 1.33 - 3.24) compared to controls. However, the test for heterogeneity was 3.43 (p value = 0.3298) indicating heterogeneity. Further details of the Asian study can be found in Table 2.

Table 2. New meta-analysis of studies investigating the association of CYP2D6 poor metaboliser genotypic polymorphisms with Parkinson's disease in Asians.

Asian Studies	Poor metaboliser (no. of patients)	OR for poor metaboliser (95% CI) [1]	Allele *CYP2D6**4	OR (95% CI) [2]
Chan/Pang et al Chinese (Hong Kong 1998) [18]				
P = 200	0	NaN	1/400	0.57
C = 227	0		2/454	(0.05-6.28)
Ho et al. Chinese (Hong Kong 1999) [66]				
P = 123		NaN	0/246	NaN
C = 124			0/248	
Woo et al Korean (2001) [67]				
P = 93	0	NaN	4/186	5.30
C = 121	0		1/244	(0.59-47.79)
Kondo/Kanazaw† Japanese (1993) [24]				
P=51	6	5.60	31/102	1.54
C=43	1	(0.65-48.48)	19/86	(0.79-2.98)
Chida et al Japanese (1999) [68]				
P = 38	0	NaN	0	NaN
C = 270	0		0	
Tsuneoka‡ et al Japanese (1998) [69]				
P = 63	7	5.56	27/126	2.83
C = 91	2	(1.12-27.73)	16/182	(1.45-5.51)

†include CYP2D6*4 or10

‡ include only CYP2D6*10, not CYP2D6*4

[1] Mantel-Haenszel odds ratio = 5.58 95% CI (1.53 - 20.33)

Test for heterogeneity: X^2 (1) = 0 (p-value = 0.9961)

[2] Mantel-Haenszel odds ratio =2.07 95% CI (1.33 - 3.24)

Test for heterogeneity: X^2 (3) = 3.43 (p-value = 0.3298)

NaN stands for "not a number", and is the result of operations such as 0/0 and Inf-Inf whose value is undefined.

CYP2D6*4, Age of Onset, PD Severity and Family History

Previous studies have suggested that CYP2D6*4 is associated with an earlier age of onset (< 50 years) of Parkinson's disease [38]. Several recent studies have addressed the relationship of CYP2D6*4 with the age of onset of Parkinson's disease and have yielded conflicting findings. Two recent studies have found no significant difference in CYP2D6*4 frequency amongst younger patients aged < 60 years [39] or aged < 50 years [40]. Both studies also failed to find a significant difference in CYP2D6*4 allele frequency when comparing Parkinson's disease patients with or without a family history of Parkinson's disease. In contrast, Payami et al [29] reported a significantly higher frequency of CYP2D6*4 in patients with late onset Parkinson's disease (age > 50 years). The authors also found a similar age-associated increase in CYP2D6*4 frequency in control subjects without Parkinson's disease and suggested that the relative CYP2D6*4 elevation in Parkinson's disease patients aged > 50 years was an age and perhaps 'survival' benefit. The CYP2D6*4 allele has been reported to be protective against cancer, especially lung cancer [26]. The enzyme is involved in the activation of procarcinogens present in tobacco smoke, and subjects who are homozygous for CYP2D6*4 may therefore be less vulnerable to the carcinogenic effect of smoking [26,41].

Stefanovic et al [42] found that the prevalence of CYP2D6*4 differed slightly in Parkinson's disease patients when compared to controls but subgroup analysis of their Parkinson's disease patients revealed that only patients with a Hoehn and Yahr staging > 2.5 had a statistically significant association. The authors suggested that the association with CYP2D6*4 was for more severe forms of Parkinson's disease and postulated that this may reflect a reduction in dopamine formation from tyramine by CYP2D6 in more advanced stages of the disease. However, the total number of patients with Parkinson's disease was small (n = 41) and the authors did not provide details of age of onset of Parkinson's disease or disease duration. Other studies have not subgrouped their Parkinson's disease cases according to different Hoehn and Yahr staging.

Limitations with Allele Association Studies

One of the most important problems of allele association studies is the lack of power due to small sample sizes. This is especially a problem when the frequency of the mutant alleles is uncommon. Frequently, even if the odds ratios are significant in some of the studies, the confidence intervals are large. Furthermore, diagnostic accuracy of Parkinson's disease remains an issue in genotypic studies using blood samples although this is overcome in a few smaller studies using brains with post mortem diagnosis showing pathological changes typical of Parkinson's disease. The clinical diagnosis of Parkinson's disease is only about 80% accurate [43]. Therefore, most of the allele studies relying on a clinical diagnosis of Parkinson's disease, may be including up to 20% of cases with other types of parkinsonism. Furthermore, the controls may also be mixed with subclinical Parkinson's disease cases.

Despite these diagnostic difficulties, which tend to underestimate positive association, a positive study will be even more positive if these biases are removed. There have been two publications, since the meta-analysis in 1998 by Christensen et al [27], comparing neuropathologically confirmed Parkinson's disease with control subjects. Atkinson et al [53], found an increased frequency of the CYP2D6*4 allele in Parkinson's disease cases confirmed neuropathologically (42% heterozygous for CYP2D6*4) when compared to controls (19% heterozygous for CYP2D6*4), although the number of Parkinson's disease cases was small (n = 33). Interestingly, the authors also compared CYP2D6*4 in neuropathologically confirmed cases of dementia with Lewy bodies and Alzheimer's disease with controls but did not find a significant association. Bon et al [44] also compared the frequency of the CYP2D6*4 and CYP2D6*3 alleles in the brains of pathologically confirmed cases of Parkinson's disease with blood samples from patients with a clinical diagnosis of parkinsonism and healthy controls. The authors found a significantly higher frequency of both alleles (35% for CYP2D6*4 and 6% for CYP2D6*3) when compared to healthy controls (19.8% for CYP2D6*4 and 3% for CYP2D6*3). They also reported an association of CYP2D6*4 with a more rapid progression (died within 10 years of diagnosis) of Parkinson's disease. However, the CYP2D6*4 allele frequency did not significantly differ between patients with a clinical diagnosis of parkinsonism and healthy controls, which the authors suggested may have been due to possible misdiagnosis of cases in the 'parkinsonism' group. In contrast, the only previous neuro-pathological study (not included in the present meta-analysis as it used archived brain tissue sample from a small number (n = 21) of neuropathologically confirmed cases of Parkinson's disease) failed to show an association with CYP2D6 [45].

Another important problem that has been ignored in allele association studies is the lack of consideration of genetic interaction with environmental factors. Both environmental and genetic factors are probably relevant in producing Parkinson's disease. A fundamental bias has been created, if one ignores the environmental factors or assumes they are the same for Parkinson's disease cases and controls in allele association studies.

Regarding the comparison of allele association studies, a number of studies have looked at CYP2D6*4 only, although there are other alleles associated with a poor metaboliser phenotype (albeit at a lower frequency). In the present meta-analysis study, the results from publications that have also compared the frequency of the CYP2D6*3 allele in Parkinson's disease patients and control subjects have been included in the final analysis. (see Table 1) In addition, due to the difference in prevalence of the mutant alleles across ethnic groups, the results may be different in different ethnic populations. In other words, if mutant alleles are infrequent in an ethnic population, even though theoretically the mutant alleles may increase an individual's risk for Parkinson's disease, at a population level, however, the increase risk may be minimal or negligible. CYP 2D6*4 polymorphism serves as a good example. It is not uncommon (5-10%) in Caucasians but very rare in Asians (< 1%). Therefore, its role in Parkinson's disease for Asians at a population level is probably not important.

Finally, a positive association in allele association studies does not imply a casual relationship, as other possibilities such as linkage disequilibrium ought to be considered.

Having listed all these problems, allele association studies remain a very useful tool in studying genetic polymorphism especially of rare diseases such as PD and may help provide a basis for more in depth studies of how a genetic defect may lead to functional deficit and disease.

Strengths and Limitations of Meta-Analysis of CYP2D6 Association with Parkinson's Disease

One way of overcoming a lack of power in allele association study is to perform studies with larger numbers or alternatively to perform a meta-analysis. Meta-analysis can overcome sample size problem and is relatively inexpensive to carry out. However meta-analysis in itself is not without problems. Publications bias exists and the potential for positive results to be preferentially published and included in the final analysis remains. Furthermore, sometimes heterogeneity may render interpretation of results difficult. Other limitations similar to allele association studies remain such as diagnostic accuracy of Parkinson's disease and lack of consideration of environmental interactions.

Review of other Susceptibility Genes

It is probable that multiple genes are involved in the pathogenesis of Parkinson's disease. Preliminary evidence of the involvement of other genes has also come from allele association studies. Generally speaking the hypothesis behind susceptibility genes is similar to CYP2D6 and usually characteristed by genetic polymorphism leading to reduced or abolished enzyme activity, and by fixed expression or homozygous allelic deletion (a theoretical correspondence between genotype and phenotype). The most commonly studied genes are those involved in oxidative stress through the generation of free radicals (phase I enzymes) or involved in scavenging (phase II enzymes) [1]. Some of the more commonly studied susceptibility genes include MAO types A (MAOA) and B (MAOB), DAT-1,dopamine receptor gene (D_2,D_3,D_4), catechol-o-methyl transferase (COMT), manganese superoxide dismutase, N-acetyltransferase 2 (NAT-2) and glutathione transferases. Results of allele association studies of PD and these susceptible genes have varied. Recently, a review of case-control studies and meta-analysis of susceptibility genes amongst Caucasians [6] has found significant associations with PD in polymorphisms of NAT-2, MAOB and GSTT1. However, all sample sizes were small with no more than 1000 cases or controls even in the meta-analysis. These studies share similar weaknesses to CYP2D6 polymorphism studies including publication bias, inherent bias of case-control studies and diagnostic accuracy of Parkinson's disease. The positive results of the meta-analysis and functions of the genes are summarized as follows:

Association of selected susceptibility genes with Parkinson's disease in Caucasians [6].

Gene	Cast/Control	Meta-analysis OR(C.I)	Possible mechanism
MAOB	204/285	2.58 (1.38-4.82)	Activate neurotoxin
NAT-2	792/912	1.33 (1.08-1.62)	Detoxify neurotoxin
tRNA Gluc	288/459	3.0 (1.1-8.2)	Mitochondrial function

Discussion

There have been many reports on the association of the poor metaboliser phenotype and genotype of CYP2D6 with Parkinson's disease. The results have been inconsistent. The major problem with most studies is that the sample size has been small which limits the statistical power. This problem can be overcome by the use of larger sample or meta-analysis. However, it should be emphasized that such an approach cannot overcome other potential methodological problems including difficulty in the diagnosis of Parkinson's disease and inherent biases of case control studies.

In this new meta-analysis, we found a small increase in the risk of PD for the poor metaboliser genotype in Caucasians but the result is only marginally significant (odds ratio = 1.36). The result of the B allele is of questionable value because of its heterogeneity and small odds ratio (1.17). Overall, one can only conclude in saying that the poor metaboliser genotype probably confers only a marginally significant genetic susceptibility to Parkinson's disease and the total percentage of patients with this risk factor is small even amongst Caucasians.

The hypothesis that mutant alleles of CYP2D6 genetic polymorphism produce poor metabolisers that fail to metabolise xenobiotics, which subsequently leads to the development of Parkinson's disease remained a plausible and attractive hypothesis. Ideally all cases and controls in allele association studies should have postmortem confirmation of pathological Parkinson's disease or the lack of it. Furthermore environmental factors should be documented and taken into account in such studies. Importantly xenobiotics exposure should be considered. Despite these shortcomings, a positive result in meta-analysis would be a more powerful clue that there is possible association of the poor metaboliser genotype of CYP2D6 and Parkinson's disease than a stand-alone smaller allele association study. If the meta-analysis result is reproducible across different ethnic groups, it will further add strength to support the hypothesis that there is an association.

In our new meta-analysis results, the Caucasian study revealed that there is an increased odds ratio or risk of Parkinson's disease in subjects who have mutant alleles producing poor metaboliser phenotypes. The situation is less clear in Asians because of the infrequency of the mutant allele. Therefore despite enlarging the sample size in the Asian meta-analysis, there is still a lack of power or sample size for a definite answer.

The fact that association studies do not imply a casual relationship should be reiterated. Other explanations including linkage disequilibrium ought to be considered. A study by Wilhelmsen et al [46] revealed that there may be two previous unknown loci near the

CYP2D6 gene that may be associated with Parkinson's disease. However these are preliminary results and no susceptibility genes have been identified at the loci mentioned.

Possible Reasons for Difference in Results between Caucasians and Asians

There are a number of possible reasons to explain the differences between Caucasian and Asian results. Firstly, although the G-to-C substitution in exon 9 at base position 4268 does not alter the activity of CYP2D6 in vitro [28], Chinese who are homozygous 4268C have a lower debrisoquine 4-hydroxylation capacity than those who are homozygous 4268G [47].

Secondly, it has been found that only 20-30% of the Japanese population that express the CYP2D6 poor metaboliser phenotype can be diagnosed by gene analysis [48]. This suggests that other possible mechanisms that control CYP2D6 gene expression could be associated with the disease outcome and may explain in part, the contradictory reports for CYP2D6 genotyping and PD.

Polymorphism of the promoter gene for CYP2D6 has been shown to alter CYP2D6 expression levels. The -1584G promoter polymorphism is associated with a statistically significantly higher expression and function of CYP2D6, than the wild type – 1584C [49]. In addition, in vitro studies have shown that the low or absent hepatic expression of CYP2D6 in HepG2 cell lines can be restored by hepatic transcription factors [50]. Similar in vitro experiments in African green monkey COS-7 cell lines have shown that hepatic nuclear factor-4α (HNF) can markedly increase CYP2D6 expression [51]. Finally through the expression of CYP2D6 activity by HNF in transgenic mice, a greater than 50% reduction in CYP2D6 activity was reported in the animals with HNF conditional mutation when compared to the control animals [52].

Conclusion

In conclusion the CYP2D6 poor metabolizer genotypes may be a putative risk factor for the pathogenesis of Parkinson's disease in Caucasians. This is supported by preliminary evidence of meta-analyses results including this latest and largest study. At a population level, this conclusion cannot be reproduced in Asians because of the rarity of the poor metabolizer genotypes amongst the Asian populations. Meta-analysis has the advantage of bigger sample size over individual allele association studies however other limitations remain. Despite extensive effort we are still left with the uncertainty about a casual relationship between CYP2D6 polymorphism and Parkinson's disease as neither meta-analysis nor individual allele association studies can prove such relationship. Further research should focus on gene-environment interactions as this will be much more meaningful than simply studying the genetic aspects or the environmental aspects separately. Because of the limitation of sample sizes it is unlikely that any single study would be able to answer the interaction question. Meta-analysis, which addresses interactions, may provide a better approach in order to answer this puzzling and interesting question.

References

[1] Chan DKY, Cordato D, Bui T, Mellick G. Comparison of environmental and genetic factors for Parkinson's disease between Chinese and Caucasians. *Neuroepidemiology* 2004; 23:13-22.

[2] Langston JW, Ballard, Tetrud JW et al. Chronic parkinsonism in humans due to a product of meperidine analog synthesis. *Science* 1983; 219:979-80.

[3] Davis GC, Williams AC, Markey SP, Ebert MH, Caine ED, Reichert EM et al. Chronic parkinsonism secondary to intravenous injection of meperidine analogues. *Psychiatry Res* 1979; 1:249-254.

[4] Calne DB, Langston JW. Etiology of Parkinson's disease. *Lancet* 1983; ii: 1457-59

[5] Kinemuchi H, Fowler CJ, TiptonKF. The neurotoxicity of 1-mthyl-4-phenyl-1,2,3,6-tetrahydropyridine (MPTP) and its relevance to Parkinson's disease. *Neurochem Int* 1987;11:359-73.

[6] Tan EK, Khajavi M, Thornby JI, Nagamitsu S, Jankovic J, Ashizawa T. Variability and validity of polymorphism association studies in Parkinson's disease. *Neurology* 2000; 55:533-538.

[7] Daily AK, Armstrong M, Monkman SC, et al. Genetic and metabolic criteria for the assignment of debrisoquine 4-hydroxylation (cytochrome P4502D6) phenotypes. *Pharmacogenetics* 1991;1:33-41.

[8] Mahgoub A, Dring LG, Idle JR, Lancaster R, Smith RL. Polymorphic hydroxylation of debrisoquine in man. *Lancet* 1977; 2:584-6.

[9] Gough AC, Miles JS, Spurr NK, et al. Identification of the primary defect at the cytochrome P450 CYP2D locus. *Nature* 1990; 347:773-76.

[10] Heim M, Meyer UA. Genotyping of poor metabolisers of debrisoquine by allele-specific PCR amplification. *Lancet* 1990; 336:529-32.

[11] Modi S, Gilham DE, Sutcliffe MJ, Lian L-Y, Primrose WU, Wolf CR, Roberts GCK: 1-methyl-4-phenyl-1,2,3,6-tetrahydropyridine as a substrate of cytochrome P450 2D6:Alosteric effects of NADPH-cytochrome P450 reuctase. *Biochemistry* 1997; 36:4461-70.

[12] Meyer UA, Zanger UM, Skoda RC, Grant D, Blum M. Genetic polymorphisms of drug metabolism. *Prog Liver Dis* 1990; 9:307-23.

[13] Relling MV. Polymorphic drug metabolism. *Clin Pharm* 1989; 8:852-63.

[14] Fonne-Pfister R, Bargetzi MJA, Meyer UA. MPTP the neurotoxin inducing Parkinson's disease, is a potent inhibitor of human and rat P450 enzymes (P450bufl, P450 adl) catalyzing debrisoquine 4-hydroxylation. *Biochem Biophys Tes. Commun* 1987; 148:1144-50.

[15] Nisnik HB, Tyndale RF, Sallee FR, et al. The dopamine transporter and cytochrome P450 2D6 (desbrisquine 4-hydroxylase) in brain: resolution and identification of two distinct [^{3}H]GBR-12935 binding proteins. *Arch Biochem Biophys* 1990; 276:424-32.

[16] Spurr NK, Gough AC, Smith CAD, Wolf CR. Genetic analysis of cytochrome P450 gene loci. *Methods Enzymol* 1991; 206:149-66.

[17] Price-Evans DA, Mihgoub A, Sloan TP, Idle JR, Smith RL. A family and population study of the genetic polymorphism of debrisoquine oxidation in a white British population. *J Med Genet* 1980; 17:102-05.

[18] Chan DKY, Woo J, Ho SC, et al. Genetic and environmental risk factors for Parkinson's disease in a Chinese population. *J Neurol Neurosurg Psychiatry* 1998; 65: 781-84.

[19] Barbeau A, Roy M, Plasse L et al. Ecogenetics of Parkinson's disease 4-hydroxylation of debrisquine. *Lancet* 1985; ii:1213-16.

[20] Kallio J, Marttila RJ, Rinne UK et al. Debrisoquine oxidation in Parkinson's disease. Acta Neurol Scand 1991; 83:194-97.

[21] Steiger MJ, Lledo P, Quinn NP et al. Debrisoquine oxidation in Parkinson's disease. *Acta Neurol Scand* 1991; 83:159-64.

[22] McCann SJ, Pond SM, James DG, et al. The association between polymorphisms in the cytochrome P-450 2D6 gene and Parkinson's disease: a case-control study and meta-analysis. *J Neurol Sci* 1997; 153:50-53.

[23] Tsuneoka Y, Matsuo Y, Iwahashi K, Takeuchi H, Ichikawa Y. A novel cytochrome P-450IID6 mutant gene associated with Parkinson's disease. J Biochem 1993; 114:263-266.

[24] Kondo I, Kanazawa I. Debrisoquine hydroxylase and Parkinson's disease. *Adv Neurol* 1993; 60:338-342.

[25] Akhmedova SN, Pushova EA, Yakimovsky AF et al. Frequency of a specific cytochrome P4502D6B (CYP2D6B) mutant allele in clinically differentiated groups of patients with Parkinson disease. *Biochemical & Molecular Medicine.* 1995; 54:88-90.

[26] Rostami-Hodjegan A, Lennard MS, Woods HF et al. Meta-analysis of studies of the CYP2D6 polymorphism in relation to lung cancer and Parkinson's disease. *Pharmacogenetics* 1998; 8:227-238.

[27] Christensen PM, GOtzsche PC, Brosen K. The sparteine/debrisoquine (CYP2D6) oxidation polymorphism and the risk of Parkinson's disease: a meta-analysis. *Pharmacogenetics* 1998; 8:227-238.

[28] Persad AS, Stedeford T, Tanaka S, Liping C, Marek B. Parkinson's Disease and CYP2D6 Polymorhisms in Asian Populations: A Meta-Analysis. *Neuroepidemiology* 2003; 22:357-361.

[29] Payami H, Lee BS, Zareparsi S, et al. Parkinson's disease, CYP2D6 polymorphism and age. *Neurology* 2001; 56:1363-1370.

[30] R is a free software distributed under a Gun-style copyleft

[31] Wolf FM. Meta-Analysis Quantitive Methods For Research Synthesis. 1986; p43, Sage Publications

[32] Becker BJ and Hedges LV. "Meta-analysis of cognitive gender difference: A comment on an analysis by Rosenthal and Rubin." *Journal of Educational Psychology* 1984; 76:583-587.

[33] Tao E, Liu Z, Chen B, Pan X, Shao M: Association between the debrisoquine hydroxylase gene polymorphism and the genetic susceptibility of Parkinson's disease. *Zhonghua Yi Xue Yi Chuan Zue Za Zhi* 1998; 15:281-283.

[34] Iwahashi K, Yoshihara E, Nakamura K, Ameno K, Watanabe M, Tsuneoka Y, Ichikawa Y, Igarashi K: CYP2D6 *HhaI* genotype and the neuroleptic malignant syndrome. *Neuropsychobiology* 1999; 39:33-37.

[35] Pang CP, Zhang J, Woo J, et al. Rarity of debrisoquine hydroxylase gene polymorphism in Chinese patients with Parkinson's disease. *Mov Disord* 1998; 13:529-32

[36] Tsuneoka Y Matsuo Y, Iwahashi K, Takeuchi H, Ichikawa Y: A novel cytochrome P-4502D6 mutant gene associated with Parkinson's disease. *J Biochem (Tokyo)* 1993; 114:263-266.

[37] Lo H-S, Chen C-H, Hogan EL, Kao K-P, Wang V, Yan S-H: Genetic polymorphism and Parkinson's disease in Taiwan: Study of debrisoquine 4-hydroxylase gene polymorphism in Chinese patients with Parkinson's disease. *Mov Disord* 1998; 13:529-532.

[38] Agundez JA, Jiminez-Jiminez FJ, Luengo A et al. Association between the oxidative polymorphism and early onset Parkinson's disease. *Clin Pharmacol Ther* 1995; 57:291-98.

[39] Sabbagh N, Brice A, Marez D, et al. CYP2D6 polymorphism and Parkinson's disease susceptibility. *Mov Disord* 1999; 14:130-136.

[40] Joost O, Taylor CA, Thomas CA, et al. Absence of effect of seven functional mutations in the CYP2D6 gene in Parkinson's disease. *Mov Disord* 1999; 14: 590-595.

[41] Vincent-Viry M, Fournier B, Galteau MM. Short communication. The effects of drinking and smoking on the CYP2D6 metabolic capacity. *Drug Metab Dispos* 2000; 28:617-619.

[42] Štefanović M, Topić E, Ivanišević A-M, Relja M, Koršić M. Genotyping of CYP2D6 in Parkinson's disease. *Clin Chem Lab Med* 2000; 38(9):929-934.

[43] Hughes AJ, Daniel Se, Kilford L, Lees AJ. Accuracy of clinical diagnosis of idiopathic Parkinson's disease: a clinico-pathological study of 100 cases. *J Neurol Neurosurg & Psychiatry* 1992; 55:181-84.

[44] Bon MAM, Jansen Steur ENH, de Vos RAI, Vermes I. Neurogenetic correlates of Parkinson's disease: apolipoprotein-E and cytochrome P450 2D6 genetic polymorphism. *Neurosci Lett* 1999; 266:149-151.

[45] Kösel S, Lücking CB, Egensperger R, Mehraein P, Graeber MB. Mitochondrial NADH dehydrogenase and CYP2D6 genotypes in Lewy-body parkinsonism. *J Neurosci Res* 1996; 44:174-183.

[46] Wilhelmsen K, Mirel D, Marder K, et al. Is there a genetic susceptibility locus for Parkinson's disease on chromosome 22q13? *Ann Neurol* 1997; 541:813-817.

[47] Wang S-L, Huang J-d, Lai M-D, Liu B-H, Lai M-L: Molecular basis of genetic variation in debrisoquin hydroxylation in Chinese subjects: Polymorphism in RFLP and DNA sequence of CYP2D6. *Clin Pharmacol Ther* 1993; 53:410-18.

[48] Yokoi T, Kosaka Y, Chida M, et al. A new CYPD2D6 allele with a ninebase insertion in exon 9 in a Japanese population associated with poor metabolizer phenotype. *Pharmacogenetics* 1996; 6:395-401.

[49] Zanger UM, Fischer J, Raimundo S, et al. Comprehensive analysis of the genetic factors determining expression and function of hepatic CYPD2D6. *Pharmacogenetics* 2001; 11:573-585.

[50] Jover R, Bort R, Gómez-Lechón MJ, Castell JV: Re-expression of C/EBPa induces CYP2B6, CYP2C9 and CYP2D6 genes in HepG2 cells. *FEBS Lett* 1998; 431:227-230.

[51] Cairns W, Smith CAD, McLaren AW, Wolf CR: Characterization of the human cytochrome P4502D6 promoter. A potential role for antagonistic interactions between members of the nuclear receptor family. *J Biol Chem* 1996; 271:25269-25276.

[52] Corchero J, Granvil CP, Feigenbaum L, Idle JR, Gonzalez FJ: The CYP2D6 humanized mouse: Effect of the human CYP2D6 transgene and HNF4a on the disposition of debrisoquine in the mouse. *Mol Phamracol* 2001; 60:1260-1267.

[53] Atkinson A, Singleton AB, Steward A, et al. CYP2D6 is associate with Parkinson's disease but not with dementia with Lewy bodies or Alzheimer's disease. *Pharmacogenetics* 1999; 9:31-35.

[54] Armstrong M, Daly AK, Cholerton S, et al. Mutant debrisoquine hydroxylation genes in Parkinson's disease. *Lancet* 1992; 339:1017-1018.

[55] Bordet R, Broly F, Destee A, Libersa C. Debrisoquine hydroxylation genotype in familial forms of idiopathic Parkinson's disease. *Adv Neurol* 1996; 36:387-396.

[56] Diederich N, Hilger C, Goetz CG, et al. Genetic variability of the CYP2D6 gene is not a risk factor for sporadic Parkinson's disease. *Ann Neurol* 1996; 40:463-465.

[57] Gasser T. Muller-Myhsok B, Supala A, et al. The CYP2D6B allele is not over represented in a population of German patients with idiopathic Parkinson's disease. *J Neurol Neurosurg Psychiatry* 1996; 61:518-519.

[58] Harhangi BS, Oostra BA, Heutink P, van Duijn CM, Hofman A, Breteler MMB. CYP2D6 polymorphism in Parkinson's disease: the Rotterdam study. *Mov Disord* 2001; 16:290-293.

[59] Kurth JH, Kurth MC, Podulso SE, et al. Association of a monoamine oxidase B allele Parkinson's disease. *Ann Neurol* 1993; 33:368-372.

[60] Lucotte G, Turpin JC, Gerard N, et al. Mutation frequencies of the cytochrome CYP2D6 gene in Parkinson disease patients and in families. *Am J Med Genet* 1996; 67(4):361-5

[61] Maraganore DM, Farrar MJ, Hardy JA, McDonnell SK, Schaid DJ, Rocca WA. Case-control study of debrisoquine-4-hydroxylase, N-acetyltransferase 2, and apolipoprotein E gene polymorphisms in Parkinson's disease. *Mov Disord* 2000; 15:714-719.

[62] Nicholl DJ, Bennett P, Hiller L, et al. A study of five candidate genes in Parkinson's disease and related neurodegenerative disorders. European Study Group on Atypical Parkinsonism. *Neurology* 1999; 53(7):1415-21

[63] Plante-Bordeneuve V, Maraganore DM, Marsden CD, et al. Debrisoquine hydrosxylase gene polymorphism in familial Parkinson's disease. *J Neurol Neurosurg Psychiatry* 1994; 57:911-3

[64] Sandy MS, Armstrong M, Tanner CM, et al. CYP2D6 allelic frequencies in young-onset Parkinson's disease. *Neurology* 1996; 47:225-30

[65] Smith CAD, Gough AC, Leigh PN, et al. Debrisoquine hydroxylase gene polymorphism and susceptibility to Parkinson's disease. *Lancet* 1992; 339:1375-1377.

[66] Ho S-L, Kung MHW, Li LSW, Lauder I, Ramsden DB. Cytochrome P4502D6 (debrisoquine 4-hydroxylase) and Parkinson's disease in Chinese and Caucasians. *Eur J Neurol* 1999; 6:323-329.

[67] Woo SIL, Kim JW, Seo HG, et al. CYP2D6*4 polymorphism is not associated with Parkison's disease and has no protective role against Alzheimer's disease in the Korean population. *Psychaitr Clin Neurosci* 2001; 55:373-377.

[68] Chida M, Hokoi T, Kosaka Y, et al. Genetic polymorphism of CYP2D6 in the Japanese population. *Pharmacogenetics* 1999; 9:601-605.

[69] Tsuneoka Y, Natsuo Y, Ichikawa Y, Watanabe Y: Genetic analysis of the CYP2D6 gene in patients with Parkinson's disease. *Mov Disord* 1998; 13:529-32.

In: Focus on Parkinson's Disease Research
Editor: Marianne J. Willow, pp. 21-43
ISBN 1-59454-924-9
© 2006 Nova Science Publishers, Inc.

Chapter II

ROLES OF CNS OXIDATION AND METHYLATION OF DOPAMINE NEUROTRANSMITTER IN PARKINSON'S DISEASE

Bao Ting Zhu[*,ϒ]
Department of Basic Pharmaceutical Sciences, College of Pharmacy,
University of South Carolina, Columbia, USA

ABSTRACT

Parkinson's disease (PD) is a common progressive neurological disorder that is characterized pathologically by the degeneration of dopaminergic neurons in the substantia nigra pars compacta (SNpc) and elsewhere. PD has multiple etiological factors, and in this article, I discussed the theoretical basis and experimental evidence for the hypothesis that dopamine oxidation in the central nervous system (CNS) plays a crucial role in the etiology of human PD. It is known that dopamine neurotransmitter is chemically reactive and its oxidation products are highly neurotoxic. Since a continual loss of SNpc dopaminergic neurons in humans is an age-dependent process and is part of the normal aging, it is theorized that PD likely is the result of an abnormal acceleration of a normal aging process, which is caused by genetic predispositions and/or various environmental factors. Specifically, a concept-building discussion of the following specific topics is provided here: (i) role of CNS dopamine oxidation in the etiology of PD; (ii) role of CNS catechol-O-methyltransferase (COMT) inadequacy in PD; (iii) serious drawbacks associated with levodopa-based pharmacotherapy of PD; (iv) usefulness of central vs. peripheral COMT inhibitors as an adjuvant in the treatment of

* Correspondence concerning this article should be addressed to Dr. Bao Ting Zhu, Department of Basic Pharmaceutical Sciences, College of Pharmacy, University of South Carolina, Room 617 of Coker Life Sciences Building, 700 Sumter Street, Columbia, SC 29208, USA. PHONE: 803-777-4802; FAX: 803-777-8356; E-MAIL: BTZhu@cop.sc.edu.

ϒ Supported in part by grants from the American Parkinson's Disease Association and the California Table Grape Commission.

PD; (v) advantages of centrally-acting, noncatechol dopamine receptor agonists in the treatment of PD; and (vi) a proposed dietary strategy for lowering the risk of PD. It is believed that the novel mechanistic understandings developed here may also offer insights into the pathogenic mechanisms of other age-dependent neurodegenerative diseases.

Keywords: Parkinson's disease; levodopa; catechol-O-methyltransferase (COMT); SAM, S-adenosyl-L-methionine; SAH, S-adenosyl-L-homocysteine.

Abbreviations

PD	Parkinson's disease
SNpc	substantia nigra pars compacta
CNS	central nervous system
COMT	catechol-O-methyltransferase
SAM	S-adenosyl-L-methionine
SAH	S-adenosyl-L-homocysteine
GSH	glutathione.

Introduction

Parkinson's disease (PD) is characterized pathologically by the degeneration of dopaminergic neurons in the substantia nigra pars compacta (SNpc) and elsewhere, typically in association with the presence of ubiquinated protein deposits in the cytoplasm of neurons (called "Lewy bodies") and thread-like proteinaceous inclusions within neurites (called "Lewy neurites") [1,2]. The current understanding of the pathophysiology of PD largely stemmed from neurochemical investigations in the 1950s–60s, with the demonstration of a >80% reduction of the striatal dopamine content along with the loss of SNpc dopaminergic neurons in most PD patients. Despite these seminal earlier findings as well as other important advances made in the ensuing decades, the exact cause for PD still eludes identification. It appears that multiple etiological factors, encompassing genetic, environmental, and intrinsic, may all play a contributing role in the development of human PD.

Over the past century, many individual cases involving apparently inherited PD in certain families had been reported in scientific literature. Studies of twins [4-7] and of families [8-12] where PD was common had led to the suggestion that some people might have an inherited susceptibility to PD. Recent studies have provided evidence for specific defects in certain genes which can lead to the development of PD in some families [reviewed in ref. 13 and 14], although these genetic abnormalities may only account for a very small fraction of all PD cases. Besides genetic factors, it has also been widely suggested that certain environmental factors may play a role in the etiology of PD. This suggestion was, in part, supported by the earlier findings that certain chemical toxins, such as N-methyl-4-phenyl-1,2,3,6-tetrahydropyridine (MPTP), could induce severe and irreversible parkinsonism in laboratory animals and humans [15-23]. Similarly, epidemiological studies by others have suggested that people with unusually high levels of pre-exposure to herbicides or pesticides were more likely to develop PD than people who did not have this exposure. However, it should be pointed out that presently there is no evidence of any kind that would suggest a widespread prior exposure of PD patients to MPTP, herbicides/pesticides, or other related chemical toxins. It is of interest to note that, besides environmental chemical toxins, PD-like symptoms had also been widely described in people who suffered a particularly severe form of influenza during an epidemic in the early 1900s.

In the past two decades, there has been some research interest in exploring a possible link between the high levels of oxidative stress detected in the SNpc and the cumulative damage in the dopaminergic neurons in PD patients [reviewed in refs. 23-26]. In this article, a particular emphasis has been placed on the conceptual development and understanding of the pathogenic changes that are indigenous to the SNpc dopaminergic neurons as an important etiological factor in human PD, on the basis of the following fundamental reasons: (i) It is well-known that dopamine neurotransmitter is chemically-reactive and its oxidation products, if formed, are highly toxic to neuronal cells. (ii) All the available studies have uniformly confirmed that the age-dependent continual loss of the SNpc dopaminergic neurons is a normal part of the aging process in humans. Although people with PD lose at least 60% (usually >80%) of their SNpc dopaminergic neurons, this likely results from an abnormal acceleration of the normal aging process, which might be affected by genetic predispositions and/or environmental factors. (iii) Almost without exceptions, PD patients that chronically receive levodopa-based therapy to alleviate symptoms would have their overall conditions markedly worsen within a few years. Notably, a recent clinical trial with pramipexole (a *noncatechol* dopamine receptor agonist) indicated that long-term use of this drug may slow the progression of PD, which is in striking contrast to the levodopa-based therapy and also suggests that the worsening of PD does not necessarily occur with all therapeutic drugs. In addition, I have also discussed in this article a large body of other experimental evidence for the proposed hypotheses/concepts, with a particular focus on the roles of CNS dopamine oxidation and COMT-mediated dopamine methylation in the etiology and prevention of human PD.

Specifically, I have provided a concept-building discussion of the following topics in this chapter: (i) role of CNS dopamine oxidation in the etiology of PD; (ii) relevance of CNS COMT inadequacy in PD; (iii) serious drawbacks associated with levodopa-based pharmacotherapy of PD; (iv) comparison of the central vs. peripheral COMT inhibitors as an adjuvant in the treatment of PD; (v) advantages of centrally-acting, noncatechol dopamine receptor agonists in the treatment of PD; and (vi) a proposed novel dietary strategy for lowering the risk of PD.

Role of CNS Dopamine Oxidation in the Etiology of PD

It is well known that the catecholamine neurotransmitters (such as dopamine and norepinephrine) in the CNS are chemically-reactive molecules. Normally, the majority (95%) of the released dopamine neurotransmitters are efficiently and quickly reuptaken into the neurons (or nerve terminals), and then further reuptaken into the storage vesicles for re-use. These reuptake processes are believed to be mediated by energy-dependent, specific membrane transportors. Although it is not known exactly what percentage of the dopamine molecules inside a neuron will be reuptaken into the storage vesicles, the fraction of the intracellular dopamine that is not reuptaken into the vesicles likely is the source that may cause cytotoxic damage to dopaminergic neurons. This suggestion appeared to be consistent with the finding that while the loss of dopaminergic neurons in the SNpc is usually drastic, there is generally no loss of neurons to a similar extent in the postsynaptic neurons in this region.

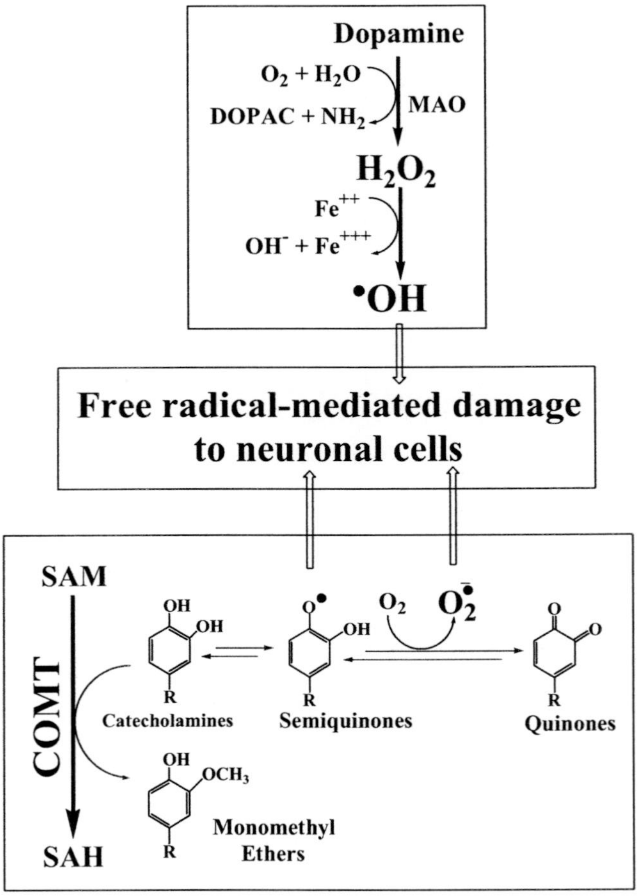

Figure 1. Contribution of different pathways of catecholamine metabolic activation to neuronal toxicity. The lower panel depicts the redox cycling between catecholamines and their semiquinone and quinone intermediates. The oxygen radicals and the catecholamine semiquinones are highly cytotoxic and also potentially genotoxic to neuronal cells. The upper panel depicts the monoamine oxidase (MAO)-mediated pathway of dopamine oxidation leading to the formation of H_2O_2 and hydroxyl radicals, which may also contribute to neuronal toxicity. DOPAC is the abbreviation for 3,4-dihyroxyphenylacetic acid, a common dopamine metabolite.

There are two major metabolic pathways by which dopamine can be oxidized, resulting in the production of oxyradicals and reactive intermediates inside a dopaminergic neuron.

One of the metabolic pathways is the oxidation of dopamine or its catechol-containing precursors and its metabolites (such as levodopa and 3,4-dihydroxyphenylacetic acid) to corresponding quinone/semiquinone intermediates [24,25] (depicted in Fig. 1). The ensuing redox cycling between the catechols and their semiquinones/quinones can continuously produce large amounts of oxyradicals. Both dopamine quinone/semiquinone intermediates and the oxygen radicals are highly cytotoxic and potentially genotoxic [25,27,28]. Notably, many different types of oxidizing enzymes (e.g., cytochrome P450 enzymes, tyrosine hydroxylase, tyrosinase, and lactoperoxidase) each can serve as efficient catalyst for the redox cycling reactions. Moreover, this process can also occur automatically in the absence of catalytic enzymes, a process commonly known as "catecholamine autooxidation".

In addition, during the monoamine oxidase (MAO)-mediated metabolic conversion of dopamine to 3,4-dihydroxyphenylacetic acid, hydrogen peroxide (H_2O_2) is generated. Hydrogen peroxide, in the presence of ferrous ion, which appears to be abundant in the SNpc neurons, may generate hydroxyl free radicals via the Fenton reaction [26], a well-known process that may further add to the free radical-mediated neuronal damage (depicted in Fig. 1). Although the potential contribution of the monoamine oxidase-mediated metabolism of dopamine to the oxidative stress in the SNpc dopaminergic neurons has received a great deal of attention in the past [23], it is possible that this pathway may be of relatively lesser importance when compared to the redox cycling between dopamine (or its catechol-containing precursors or metabolites) and the corresponding semiquinone/quinone intermediates. Somewhat in line with this suggestion, an earlier large clinical trial has shown that the monoamine oxidase inhibitor selegiline had little or no neuroprotective effect in PD patients [29], although more studies would be necessary to confirm this observation and also to compare the protective effects of different antioxidants in human PD.

I have briefly discussed below several lines of experimental evidence from both animal and human studies which provides considerable support for the hypothesis that the oxidative damage caused by free radicals and reactive dopamine intermediates is an important indigenous etiological factor in human PD:

(1) There are consistent data showing that the brain SNpc region of PD patients had elevated levels of oxidative stress, as evidenced by high levels of oxidation products formed from lipids [30-32], proteins [33], and DNA [34].

Marked decrease (40-50%) of glutathione (GSH) content has been observed in the SNpc of PD patients [35,36]. Although earlier studies suggested that the decrease of glutathione content in the SNpc itself did not cause PD, it did provide a reliable indication for the elevated levels of oxidative stress in the affected neurons. It is of interest to point out that the decrease of glutathione levels in the SNpc of PD patients was not accompanied by increased levels of glutathione disulfide [36-38]. This observation raised the possibility that the decrease of glutathione levels might be largely due to the formation of conjugates between glutathione and reactive dopamine intermediates in the SNpc. More studies are needed to further determine this possibility.

It is also known that total iron content is increased but ferritin content is decreased in the SNpc of PD patients [39]. This combination suggests that a larger fraction of this transition metal is in an active form capable of catalyzing nonenzymatic oxidative reactions, especially the conversion of hydrogen peroxide to hydroxyl radical, which is probably the most reactive of the oxygen radicals. It has been suggested that neuromelanin, a product of dopamine autooxidation, might serve as a reservoir for iron, promoting the generation of oxyradicals. Moreover, earlier studies also showed that the activities of glutathione peroxidase and catalase in the SNpc were decreased, likely suggesting a compromised antioxidant defense mechanism in this region.

(2) Studies have suggested that neurotoxic chemicals, such as 6-hydroxydopamine and 1-methyl-4-phenyl-1,2,3,6-tetrahydropyridine (MPTP) that selectively destroyed the dopaminergic neurons in the SNpc, act through increasing the oxidative damage in these neurons [25,26]. One of the well-known effects of MPTP is the disruption of mitochondrial energy production in the SNpc neurons. It is possible that when the cellular energy production is disrupted, the released dopamine cannot be efficiently reuptaken into the storage vesicles. Moreover, large amounts of dopamine may leak out of the vesicles into the cytosolic compartment because of the disruption of the cellular energy production. All these changes would contribute to increased intracellular and extracellular accumulation of dopamine in the SNpc, and subsequently result in increased formation of free radicals and reactive dopamine intermediates inside the neurons and also within the synaptic cleft. Animal studies have shown that the glial cells in the SNpc region release large amounts of glutathione following MPTP treatment, and it is possible that the released glutathione is mainly to provide protection against the increased synaptic concentrations of dopamine and its reactive intermediates.

(3) It is known that 80-90% of the dopaminergic neurons are usually lost in PD patients. It should be noted that progressive loss of dopaminergic neurons, usually to a much lesser degree, is a common phenomenon during the normal course of aging. The cause for the cumulative loss of dopaminergic neurons in the SNpc during aging likely is due to the high basal levels of oxidative stress that is indigenous to these neuronal cells. Conceivably, if a person is at an abnormally high rate for losing dopaminergic neurons during the course of aging, this person may be expected to have an elevated risk for developing PD. On the other hand, the use of effective means (such as dietary supplements) that can partially protect the SNpc neurons from oxidative damage and neuronal loss may significantly reduce the risk for developing PD (discussed later).

It has been noted that extensive and widespread oxidative damage was seen in the SNpc as well as other brain regions of PD patients chronically treated with large doses of levodopa. It has been suspected that much of the observed extensive neuronal damage was caused by the prooxidant effects of the administered levodopa [40,41]. These clinical observations not only raised serious questions about the long-term therapeutic benefits of levodopa-based pharmacotherapy (more discussion is provided in later sections), but they also provided support for the hypothesis that elevated dopamine oxidation in the CNS likely is an important etiological factor in PD.

(4) Human SNpc neurons appear to contain very low levels of COMT, an important enzyme that detoxifies catecholamines in the CNS (discussed in the ensuing sections). This observation suggests that the intrinsic oxidative damage in SNpc neurons, when coupled with the low capacity for metabolic detoxification of catecholamines, may jointly contribute to the development of PD.

In summary, there is a considerable body of experimental evidence that supports the proposed hypothesis that the indigenious oxidative damage caused by dopamine oxidation is an important etiological factor in PD. More studies are urgently needed to further test this hypothesis. These studies will not only provide a better mechanistic understanding of the pathogenesis of PD as well as other age-related neurodegenerative diseases (such as Huntington's disease), but they may also lead to the development of new ways to effectively retard the development and progression of these debilitating conditions.

Relevance of CNS COMT Inadequacy in PD

Catecholamine neurotransmitters are rapidly metabolized by catecholamine-specific enzymes (namely, COMT and monoamine oxidase) as well as other nonspecific conjugating enzymes (such as sulfotransferases and glutathione S-transferases) in the CNS [42]. These metabolic pathways collectively provide effective detoxification of catecholamines and their catechol-containing precursors/metabolites, thereby preventing them from causing cytotoxic neuronal damage in the first place.

However, under certain conditions where increased amounts of oxyradicals and reactive semiquinone/quinone intermediates are formed from catecholamine neurotransmitters, a number of cellular mechanisms may step in to limit the extent of oxidative neuronal damage in certain regions of the CNS. The presence of reducing compounds, such as ascorbate (vitamin C), and the protective enzymes, such as superoxide dismutase that catalyzes the reduction of superoxide radicals, may jointly provide protection against the oxidative stress caused by elevated levels of oxyradicals. On the other hand, the presence of glutathione and glutathione-S-transferases may provide protection against the strong cytotoxicity of dopamine semiquinone/quinone intermediates.

Here I like to point out that among the metabolic detoxification pathways for catecholamines and various protective mechanisms for chemically-reactive intermediates, the COMT-mediated O-methylation of catecholamines is of unique importance. This metabolic pathway provides an efficient first-line detoxification, quickly rendering catecholamine neurotransmitters and their catechol-containing precursors/metabolites biologically inactive and chemically inert. If and when the COMT activity in the SNpc neurons becomes significantly inadequate because of inherited deficiency or due to chronic inhibition resulting from conditions such as hyperhomocysteinemia (discussed later), then dopamine and its catechol-containing precursors/metabolites cannot be rapidly deactivated by the methylation metabolism. Consequently, the concentrations of catecholamines within the SNpc dopaminergic neurons would increase, and the metabolic formation of oxyradicals and chemically-reactive semiquinone/quinone intermediates would be markedly augmented, resulting in chronic oxidative stress and possibly damage to neuronal cells [26]. Since these metabolic reactions take place mostly within the catecholaminergic neurons (e.g., SNpc dopminergic neurons), characteristic neurodegenerative damage is also expected to be seen largely within these neurons.

Summarized below are some of the experimental observations that support a protective role of the COMT-mediated methylation of dopamine in SNpc neurons:

(1) Biochemical studies have shown that COMT activity is present in the homogenates or subcellular fractions prepared from various parts of the brain. Interestingly, an earlier study by Kastner et al. [43] showed that COMT immunostaining was not detected in melanized dopaminergic neurons in human SNpc (post mortem), although dense staining was found in dopaminergic neurons in the ventral tegmental area and substantia nigra pars lateralis. Also, little COMT immunostaining was seen in dopaminergic nerve terminals in connection with the striatal dendritic spines, whereas COMT immunostaining was found in numerous cell bodies and in neuropiles in the striatum.

The observations by Kastner et al. [43] are very intriguing, and more studies are needed to confirm these important findings and extend the conclusions. It will be of interest to determine if this is a general age-related phenomenon in humans. There may be good explanations for the above observations: First, the total population of dopaminergic neurons left in the SNpc of an elderly person likely is very low, resulting from the continuous loss of dopaminergic neurons in this region during the normal course of aging. Second, the SNpc dopaminergic neurons may contain indigenously lower levels of COMT when compared to other dopaminergic neurons in the CNS. If this proves to be true, then it would clearly suggest that the SNpc dopaminergic neurons may be less protected with regard to the oxidative damage caused by dopamine oxidation, and this could be an important intrinsic factor that makes the SNpc neurons more vulnerable to dopamine-mediated damage.

(2) In a recent preliminary study by Werner et al. [44], it was found that levodopa was highly neurotoxic in cultured rat mesencephalic dopaminergic neurons. Interestingly, the presence of SAM (the direct methyl donor for COMT-mediated methylation) or methionine or dimethionine (precursors for the biosynthesis of SAM) each protected these neurons from the damage induced by levodopa. Moreover, their protective effect against levodopa's neuronal toxicity was essentially abolished when a COMT inhibitor was present. These preliminary observations are consistent with the important protective role of the COMT metabolic pathway in SNpc neurons.

(3) It was recently postulated that hyperhomocysteinemia can lead to inhibition of COMT-mediated methylation of catecholamines as well as other catechol substrates [45,46]. Homocysteine, a sulfur-containing amino acid normally present at low concentrations in blood and cells, is an intermediate involved in the biosynthesis and metabolism of methionine, cysteine, SAM, and SAH. Inside a cell, SAH is recycled to form SAM via enzymatic conversion first to homocysteine and then to methionine as intermediates (depicted in Fig. 2). The conversion of SAH to homocysteine is catalyzed by SAH hydrolase, and the further conversion of homocysteine to methionine is mainly catalyzed by 5-homocysteine methyltransferase using vitamin B_{12} and folate as key cofactors [47]. Homocysteine can also react with serine to form cystathionine and further to cysteine, reactions that are vitamin B_6-dependent [47].

When homocysteine (or adenosine) accumulates inside the cell or after increased intake of exogenous homocysteine (or adenosine), the reaction catalyzed by SAH hydrolase will be directed toward SAH biosynthesis, with concomitant reduction in the enzymatic degradation of SAH. Consequently, high cellular levels of SAH will result. This has been demonstrated in cultured or isolated cells [48-51], in perfused liver or heart [52,53], and in whole animals [54,55]. As discussed earlier, elevated levels of SAH resulting from hyperhomocysteinemia would noncompetitively inhibit the COMT-mediated O-methylation of endogenous catecholamines as well as other catechol substrates, subsequently resulting in accumulation of catecholamine neurotransmitters and causing oxidative damage to cells that are exposed to elevated concentrations of catecholamines. In the case of dopaminergic neurons, hyperhomocysteinemia is expected to increase their oxidative damage and thus would be a specific risk factor for PD.

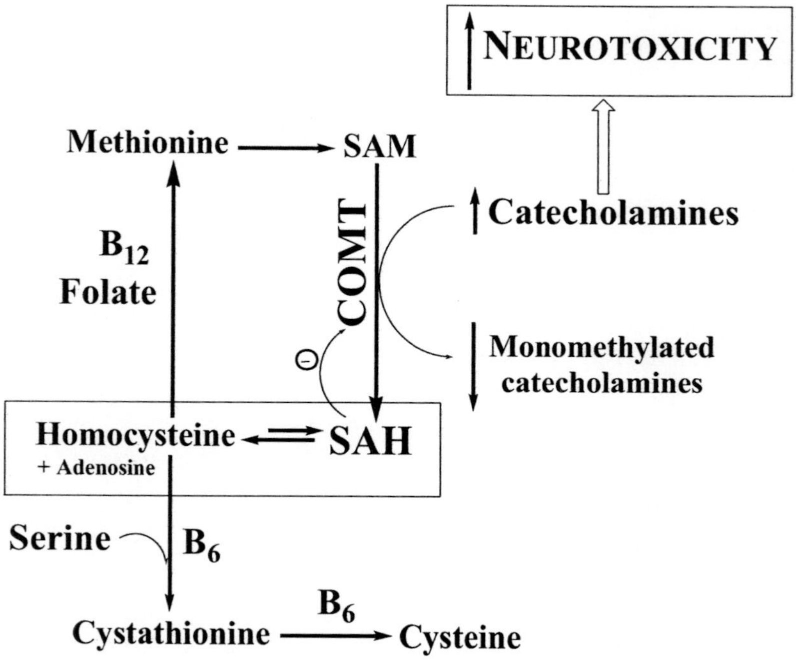

Figure 2. Proposed mechanism of homocysteine pathophysiology based on accumulation of intracellular SAH. SAH can strongly and noncompetitively inhibit COMT-mediated O-methylation of catecholamine neurotransmitters [80-82]. Inhibition of the O-methylation of catecholamines by SAH would result in their accumulation within the neuronal cells. In addition, elevated levels of catecholamines may lead to strong cytotoxicity due to formation of catechol quinone/semiquinone intermediates and oxyradicals. As shown, folate, B_6, and B_{12} are key cofactors for the major metabolic pathways that are involved in the regulation of the cellular levels of homocysteine and SAH. The presence of adequate amounts of intracellular folate, B_6 and B_{12} would be beneficial for reducing homocysteine levels through various catabolic pathways (described in detail in the text), and ultimately, reducing the intracellular levels of homocysteine and SAH.

This mechanistic explanation logically leads to the suggestion that adequate dietary intake of vitamin B_6, B_{12}, and folate may have a partial protective effect against the neuronal damage associated with hyperhomocysteinemia. As depicted in Fig. 2, vitamin B_{12} and folate are key cofactors for the enzymatic conversion of homocysteine to methionine and further to SAM. When their cellular supply is inadequate, the enzymatic conversion of homocysteine to methionine will be reduced, leading to accumulation of homocysteine plus decreased synthesis of SAM. Similarly, decreased conversion of homocysteine to cysteine (a vitamin B_6-dependent pathway, Fig. 2) also leads to accumulation of homocysteine. Elevated levels of homocysteine would inhibit the enzymatic conversion of SAH to homocysteine and consequently result in SAH accumulation. Elevated concentrations of SAH or decreased availability of SAM or combination of both would significantly slow down COMT-mediated O-methylation of endogenous catecholamines. On the other hand, supplementing exogenous vitamin B_{12} and/or folate would facilitate the conversion of homocysteine to methionine, and consequently they would decrease the levels of SAH and also increase the formation of SAM; supplementing vitamin B_6 would accelerate the conversion of homocysteine to cystathionine and cysteine, a diverging pathway that would help reduce homocysteine and SAH accumulation and thereby also partially alleviate the problem (see Fig. 2).

The above explanations are in accord with the findings from many epidemiological studies [56-59] showing that the plasma homocysteine concentrations correlated negatively with the plasma levels of folate, vitamins B_6 and B_{12}, and also correlated negatively with the dietary intake of these vitamins. It was found that hyperhomocysteinemia sensitized mice to MPTP-induced dopaminergic neurodegeneration and motor dysfunction [60]. Similarly, animals with low folate levels developed severe PD-like symptoms, while those with normal levels remained healthy [61].

(4) While we are pondering the etiological roles of CNS dopamine oxidation and COMT inadequacy in PD, an interesting question always comes to mind: Why do the medullar cells of the adrenal gland that contain even larger amounts of catecholamines (mainly epinephrine) usually not develop a similar degree of cellular damage as seen in the SNpc dopaminergic neurons? One of the explanations may lie in the fact that the adrenal medullar cells usually only release epinephrine into the circulation as a neurohormone, and these cells normally do not need to continuously reuptake epinephrine back into the cells for reuse. Consequently, these cells would have much less chance of suffering intracellular oxidative damage than the SNpc dopaminergic neurons. Furthermore, it is known that very high levels of the COMT activity are present in the adrenal medulla, which may provide effective metabolic protection against catecholamines.

In summary, the COMT-mediated methylation metabolism of endogenous catecholamines is believed to be an important first-line detoxification pathway that effectively renders them biologically inactive and chemically inert, and thereby provides protection against the potential neuronal damage caused by the subsequent oxidative metabolism of these catechols. When the methylation metabolism is compromised, the risk for developing PD may be significantly increased. Notably, an earlier study has suggested that the COMT levels in the SNpc dopaminergic neurons likely are indigenously low [43]. If this finding is confirmed in future larger scale studies, the low COMT activity in SNpc neurons could be a crucial intrinsic factor predisposing the SNpc neurons vulnerable to the damage caused by catecholamine oxidation. In addition, because hyperhomocysteinemia can lead to increased levels of SAH and subsequently inhibit the metabolic O-methylation of catecholamines, I believe that increased dietary intake of SAM (the methyl donor for COMT) along with vitamins B_6, B_{12} and folate may partially reduce the risk for developing PD in high risk populations.

SERIOUS DRAWBACKS ASSOCIATED WITH LEVODOPA-BASED PHARMACOTHERAPY OF PD

There is no cure for PD at the present time. When the patients are only mildly affected, they usually need no drug treatment for several years following the initial diagnosis. When the symptoms progress to a rigid, akinetic state in which patients are unable to care for themselves, then they are usually prescribed the levodopa-based pharmacotherapy [62,63]. Levodopa itself is largely inactive pharmacologically, and its therapeutic and adverse effects result from decarboxylation of levodopa to dopamine. Clinical studies have shown that levodopa-based therapy can markedly improve the symptoms of PD. Notably, the duration of the beneficial effects of levodopa in early stages of PD usually exceeds the plasma lifetime of the drug, suggesting that the nigrostriatal dopamine system still retains some capacity to store and release dopamine. Following chronic use of levodopa, however, this apparent buffering capacity gradually disappears, and the patient's motor state usually starts to fluctuate dramatically with each dose of levodopa. A common problem is the development of the so-called "wearing-off" phenomenon, which usually means that each dose of levodopa effectively improves mobility for a short period of time (perhaps 1-2 hours), but rigidity and akinesia rapidly return at the end of the dosing interval. Increasing the dose and frequency of administration can improve this situation, but this is often limited by the development of dyskinesias (excessive and abnormal involuntary movements). These movements can be equally uncomfortable and disabling as PD-caused rigidity and akinesia. In later stages of PD, patients may suffer from rapid fluctuations between being "off" (having no beneficial effects from their medications) and being "on" but with disabling dyskinesias. Because of these uncertainties, most practitioners have adopted a pragmatic approach, using levodopa only when the symptoms of PD cause functional impairment. Nevertheless, at present levodopa is still generally considered as the most effective agent and the gold standard drug therapy for PD.

Here an important, yet still unanswered, question remains: Does chronic use of levodopa accelerate the course of PD while it modifies the symptoms only for a short term? This question is raised on the basis of the following considerations: First, if the production of free radicals and neurotoxic intermediates as a result of dopamine oxidation contributes significantly to the death of SNpc neurons, then chronic administration of large doses of levodopa would inevitably accelerate free radical-mediated neuronal degeneration. Some researchers may argue that presently there is no convincing evidence for this suggestion. It should be noted, however, that the lack of direct evidence is, in part, due to the fact that there were very few carefully-designed studies to specifically address this important medical issue. Besides, the lack of evidence somehow also reflects a sense of muted reluctance in the medical community to seriously confront the dejecting possibility that levodopa (considered to be the gold standard drug therapy) may only alleviate PD symptoms for a short term at the expense of accelerating the course of the disease. Second, if we take a careful inspection of all available clinical observations, it is very clear that the undesirable "on/off" fluctuations and the "wearing off" phenomena are almost exclusively seen in patients treated chronically with levodopa. Although there is no definitive evidence at present that would enable us to tell whether delaying the treatment with levodopa would delay the appearance of these effects, it is of note that recent clinical studies have indicated that long-term use of pramipexole and ropinrole (two noncatechol dopamine receptor agonists) might slow the progression of human PD [reviewed in refs. 64,65]. These studies suggested that the conditions of human PD may not necessarily progressively worsen with any types of drug therapy. Therefore, when all the available clinical findings are taken into consideration, the picture becomes rather clear that chronic use of large doses of levodopa accelerates the progression of human PD.

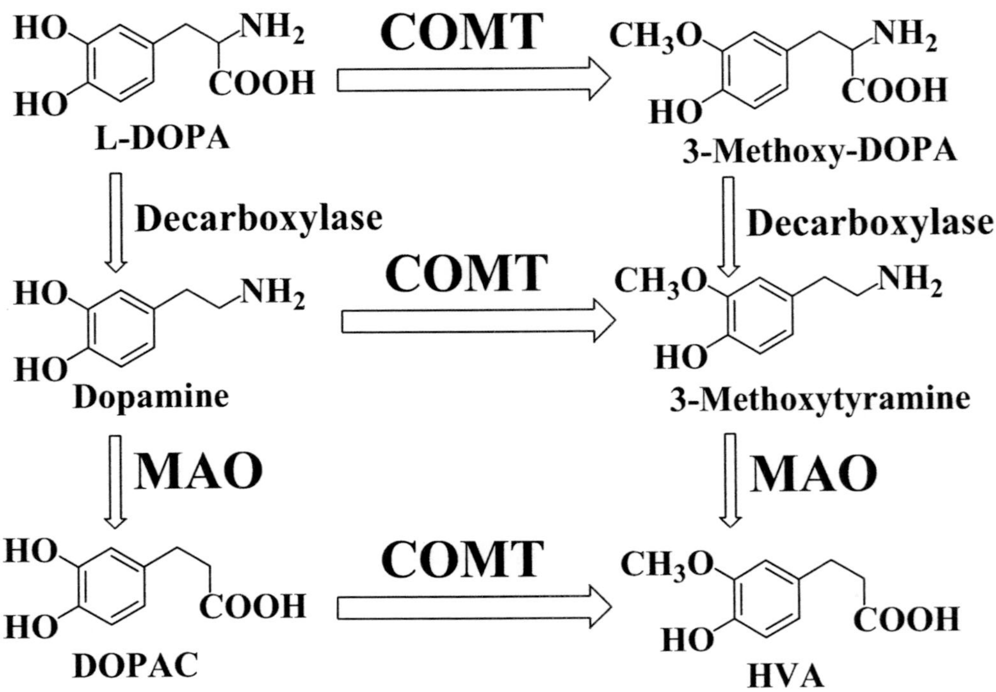

Figure 3. Roles of COMT inhibition in levodopa-based pharmacotherapy of PD. The main benefits of a peripheral inhibition of COMT-mediated methylation of levodopa include an increased bioavailability and reduced concentration fluctuations of levodopa in the CNS. In comparison, since the physiological effects of levodopa in the CNS mainly rely on vesicular release of dopamine, COMT inhibition in the CNS may not significantly alter the physiological actions of levodopa and dopamine, but it may substantially increase their neurotoxicity (due to inhibition of their major detoxification pathway).

The Benefits of Using Peripheral COMT Inhibitors as an Adjunct in Levodopa-Based Treatment of PD

In modern medicine, levodopa is always administered in combination with a peripherally-acting inhibitor of the aromatic L-amino acid decarboxylase, such as carbidopa or benserazide (Fig. 3). If levodopa is administered alone, the drug is largely decarboxylated in the intestinal mucosa and other peripheral sites, and only a very small fraction (usually <1%) of the parent drug can reach the CNS. It is also known that when dopa decarboxylase is strongly inhibited by carbidopa, the majority of the administered levodopa is then metabolized by the peripheral COMT, and 3-methyldopa becomes the major metabolite [66-

71] (Fig. 3). Accordingly, concomitant use of a selective COMT inhibitor to reduce the peripheral methylation metabolism of levodopa has been recommended to enhance levodopa's therapeutic effectiveness. A series of new and highly selective COMT inhibitors (nitrocatechol-type compounds) have already been developed for this particular purpose [72]. These compounds, through tight-binding inhibition of the COMT, effectively inhibit the O-methylation of levodopa, improve its bioavailability, and potentiate its therapeutic effects in vivo [72-76].

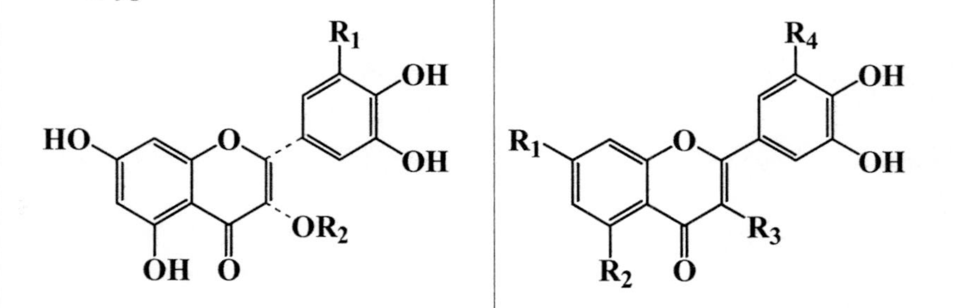

EXAMPLES	R_1	R_2	EXAMPLES	R_1	R_2	R_3	R_4
(-)-Epicatechin	-H	-H	Quercetin	-OH	-OH	-OH	-H
(+)-Epicatechin	-H	-H	Fisetin	-H	-OH	-OH	-H
(-)-Epigallocatechin	-OH	-H	Luteolin	-OH	-OH	-H	-H
(-)-Epicatechin gallate	-H	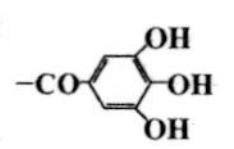	Rhamnetin	$-OCH_3$	-OH	-OH	-H
(-)-Epigallocatechin gallate	-H	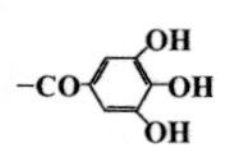	Myricetin	-OH	-OH	-OH	-OH

Figure 4. Structures of representative polyphenolic dietary compounds that are excellent substrates and inhibitors of the COMT-mediated O-methylation metabolism. Note that these polyphenolic compounds all have a catechol structure. Most of these polyphenolic compounds are richly present in our diet, such as tea, orange juice, grapes, onions, and chocolates.

Presently, two COMT inhibitors (tolcapone and entacapone) are available for human use in the United States. Clinical studies with PD patients receiving levodopa plus carbidopa showed that entacapone and tolcapone prolonged the therapeutic effectiveness of levodopa, and they also reduced, to varying degrees, the "wearing-off" symptoms in these patients [77]. Although the mechanisms of action of these COMT inhibitors are similar, they differ in their pharmacokinetic properties. Tolcapone has a relatively long duration of action, allowing for administration 2 to 3 times a day, and is believed to act through inhibiting both central and peripheral COMT. In comparison, the action of entacapone is short, ~2 hrs, and it is usually administered simultaneously with each dose of levodopa/carbidopa. The action of entacapone is believed to be attributable principally to its inhibition of the peripheral COMT.

It should be noted that in recent years some researchers have suggested that COMT inhibitors with preferential CNS activity would have more desirable therapeutic benefits than those inhibitors with preferential peripheral activity. This strategy may prove to be incorrect in light of the possibility that the oxidative intermediates generated from dopamine/levodopa oxidation within the SNpc may aggravate neurodegenerative damage. Instead, it is reasonable to suggest that COMT inhibitors with selective peripheral activity would be more desirable than those with strong central effects. Strong inhibition of the central COMT would facilitate the oxidative damage stemming from the accumulation of levodopa and dopamine and their subsequent oxidation in certain brain regions. In comparison, selective inhibition of peripheral COMT would effectively increase the bioavailability of levodopa in the CNS through inhibition of its peripheral methylation metabolism, leaving mostly intact the COMT-mediated protective metabolism in the CNS (explained in Fig. 3).

It is of note that Zhu et al. have observed that several catechol-containing dietary phytochemicals (such as bioflavonoids and tea catechins; structures shown in Fig. 4) were exceptionally good substrates for the COMT-mediated O-methylation metabolism [78-82]. Recent additional studies also showed that these dietary polyphenols are effective inhibitors of the COMT-mediated O-methylation of some catechol substrates [Fig. 5; ref. 83]. Since these polyphenolic phytochemicals are highly water-soluble and usually largely remain in the peripheral compartment, it will be of considerable interest to determine whether these dietary chemicals can beneficially inhibit the peripheral methylation metabolism of levodopa. These water-soluble phytochemicals may constitute a new class of nontoxic dietary inhibitors of COMT with a predominant peripheral activity.

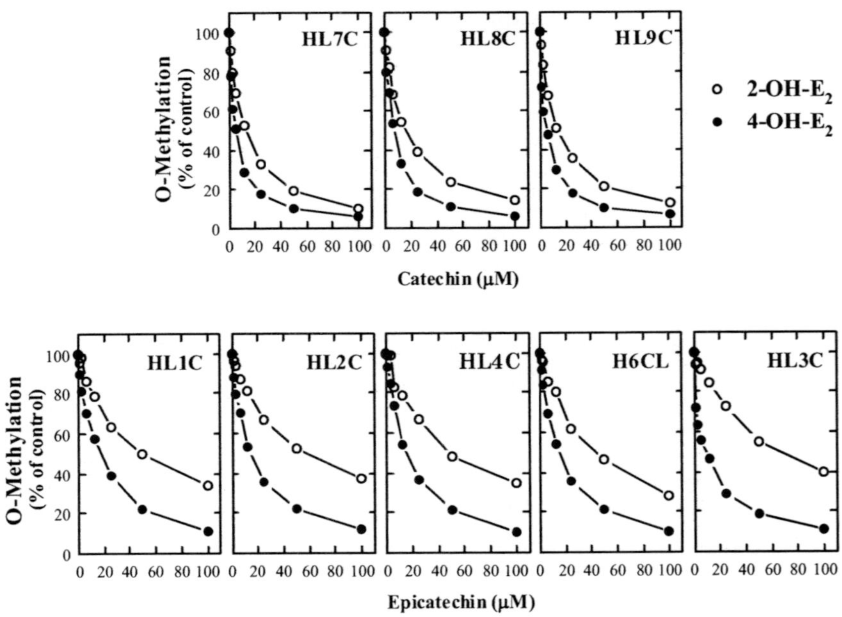

Figure 5. Inhibition of human liver COMT-mediated O-methylation of 2- and 4-hydroxyestradiol (2-OH-E_2 and 4-OH-E_2, respectively) by different concentrations of catechin and epicatechin. The reaction conditions were described in ref. [83]. The incubation mixture consisted of 10 μM of 2-OH-E_2 or 4-OH-E_2, 250 μM [^{3}H-methyl]S-adenosyl-L-methionine (containing 0.2 μCi), 0.5 mg/ml of human liver cytosolic protein, 1 mM dithiothreitol, and 1.2 mM $MgCl_2$ in a final volume of 0.25 ml reaction buffer (10 mM, pH 7.4). Incubations were carried out at 37°C for 10 min. Each point is the mean of duplicate determinations (with average variations <5%).

ADVANTAGES OF CENTRALLY-ACTING, NONCATECHOL DOPAMINE RECEPTOR AGONISTS FOR THE TREATMENT OF PD

As a promising alternative to levodopa-based therapy of PD, the use of non-catechol dopamine agonists to selectively activate the postsynaptic striatal dopamine receptors has recently received a great deal of attention. Here it should be emphasized that from both theoretical and pharmacotherapeutic points of view, the use of centrally-acting, non-catechol dopamine agonists would not only provide alleviation of the clinical symptoms, but these agents would also have many potential advantages over levodopa-based therapy. First, since enzymatic conversion of these drugs is not required for therapeutic actions, their effectiveness is not dependent on the functional capacity of the nigrostriatal neurons, and thus they could be more useful than levodopa for the treatment of late-stage PD. Second, selective dopamine receptor agonists could have more selective actions than levodopa (a precursor of dopamine), because the latter can nonselectively activate all dopamine receptor subtypes in the brain. In this context, it should be pointed out that an ideal dopamine receptor agonist for the treatment of PD would be the one that can selectively activate the postsynaptic striatal dopamine receptor subtype(s) to effectively elicit its therapeutic effects, but hopefully it would not activate the presynaptic dopamine receptors that may inhibit the physiological release of endogenous dopamine neurotransmitter from the SNpc. Further along this line of thought, it may be even more desirable if the dopamine receptor agents are bifunctional agents that could not only selectively activate the postsynaptic dopamine receptors, but could also simultaneously antagonize the presynaptic dopamine autreceptors in the SNpc (which would lead to enhanced physiological release of the endogenous dopamine neurotransmitter). The proposed properties of an ideal dopamine receptor agent for PD are depicted in Fig. 6. Third, dopamine agonists could have duration of action much longer than levodopa and thus could make them more useful in the management of dose-related fluctuations in motor states. Lastly, and most importantly, in light of the known neurotoxic effects of reactive quinone/semiquinone intermediates of levodopa and dopamine and various derived free radicals, the use of *noncatechol* dopamine agonists may effectively slow down the progression and aggravation of PD while providing alleviation of clinical symptoms.

It is of note that the two prototypic dopamine receptor agonists, bromocriptine and pergolide (both are ergot derivatives), have already been in clinical use for PD for quite some time. Bromocriptine is a strong agonist of the dopamine D_2 receptor and a partial antagonist of the D_1 receptor, while pergolide acts as an agonist at both D_1 and D_2 receptor subtypes. The overall therapeutic actions as well as the side effects of these two drugs appear to be quite similar to those of levodopa. Their duration of action after a single dose often is longer than that of levodopa, and thus a lessening of "on/off" fluctuations can be observed. According to the proposed requirements for an ideal dopamine receptor agent for the treatment of PD (depicted in Fig. 6), it is apparent that these two agents are far from ideal because they are not preferentially active for the postsynaptic dopamine receptors (mainly D_1) over presynaptic dopamine autoreceptors (mainly D_2).

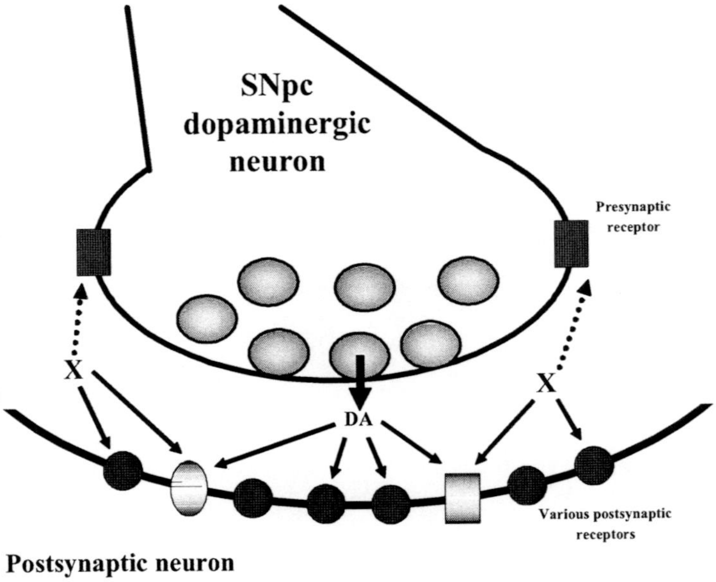

Figure 6. Proposed ideal dopamine receptor agent for the treatment of human PD. As depicted, an ideal agent (X) should be a bifunctional agent that would not only selectively activate the postsynaptic dopamine receptors, but could also simultaneously block the presynaptic dopamine autoreceptors in the SNpc. Antagonism of these presynaptic receptors would lead to enhanced release of endogenous dopamine neurotransmitters, which would be greatly beneficial in PD patients.

Notably, several new dopamine receptor agonists, such as pramipexole and ropinirole, recently also became available for clinical use in PD. Interestingly, clinical studies have suggested that pramipexole might slow the progression of PD, and similar results were also observed with ropinirole. These findings are very exciting, although more studies are warranted to further confirm these findings. Their apparent superior therapeutic profile may be largely related to their differential activity at the postsynaptic dopamine receptors vs. presynaptic receptors at the SNpc. Because of the multitude of potential advantages associated with noncatechol dopamine agonists in the treatment of PD (discussed above), it is hoped that more selective dopamine agonists will be designed in the future for testings in animal models and humans so that a better alternative pharmacotherapy for PD may be rationally developed.

Proposed Dietary Strategy to Lower the Risk of Human PD

On the basis of the novel mechanistic understanding developed here, I propose a dietary strategy that is tailored toward reducing the risk factors associated with human PD:

(1) To enhance the COMT-mediated O-methylation metabolism of endogenous catecholamines, dietary supplementation of SAM is recommended. Similarly, to lower the blood levels of homocysteine (particularly in the case of hyperhomocysteinemia) and also to

accelerate the biosynthesis of endogenous SAM, it is recommended to take adequate amounts of vitamin B_6, B_{12}, and folate. Adequate intake of these vitamins would not only reduce the risk of various cardiovascular diseases [discussed in refs. 45,46], but it would also reduce the risk of neurodegenerative diseases, particularly PD. Notably, recent studies have already suggested hyperhomocysteinemia sensitizes the animals to MPTP-induced dopaminergic neurodegeneration and motor dysfunction, and animals with low folate levels developed severe PD-like symptoms, while those with normal levels remained healthy.

(2) To better protect against the reactive catecholamine intermediates and free radicals, adequate dietary supplementation of vitamin C (ascorbic acid) would be beneficial. It should be noted that although some earlier studies once suggested that high doses of vitamin E might delay the onset of severe PD symptoms, this effect had not been borne out in later clinical trials. Vitamin C may have a more effective protection than vitamin E because the former is highly water-soluble and thus would have a similar intracellular distribution that would favor the protection against the water-soluble catecholamine reactive intermediates. Interestingly, there are clinical trials also testing the PD-protecting effects of dietary supplementation of coenzyme Q_{10}, a powerful antioxidant that is thought to help protect from the mitochondrial damage often associated with PD. Its effectiveness remains to be seen.

(3) It has been widely recommended that a nutritionally-balanced diet that contains plenty of fruits, vegetables, and whole grains is beneficial for reducing the risk of PD. These food components generally contain many natural antioxidants (in addition to fiber) that may help protect against free radical-mediated damage. However, caution is advised since many types of fruits contain large amounts of polyphenols, and many of these dietary chemicals (such as flavonoids and catechins; structures shown in Fig. 4) were found to be exceptionally good substrates as well as inhibitors of COMT [78-82], which could inhibit the O-methylation of catecholamine neurotransmitters. Accordingly, the overall beneficial or harmful effects of eating excessive amounts of fruits on PD remain to be further evaluated.

Concluding Remarks

PD, a common progressive neurological disorder, has multiple etiological factors. In this article, I have discussed the theoretical basis and experimental evidence for the hypothesis that CNS dopamine oxidation plays a crucial role in the etiology of human PD. It is widely known that dopamine neurotransmitter is chemically-reactive and its oxidation products are highly neurotoxic. Since the continual loss of SNpc dopaminergic neurons in humans is an age-dependent process and is part of the normal aging, it is theorized that PD likely is the result of an abnormal acceleration of a normal aging process, which is caused by genetic predispositions and/or various environmental factors. In partial support of this hypothesis, it is almost without exceptions that PD patients who chronically receive levodopa-based therapy for alleviation of symptoms have their overall conditions markedly worsen within a few years.

I have also discussed the unique importance of COMT-mediated methylation metabolism of catecholamine neurotransmitters in their detoxification. When the methylation metabolism is compromised, the risk for developing PD may be significantly increased. Notably, an earlier study has suggested that the COMT levels in human SNpc dopaminergic neurons likely are indigenously low [43], which could be a crucial intrinsic factor predisposing these neurons vulnerable to the damage caused by catecholamine oxidation. In addition, hyperhomocysteinemia can lead to increased levels of SAH, which could subsequently inhibit the O-methylation metabolism of catecholamines.

I have also critically evaluated the overall usefulness of levodopa-based therapy of PD. Based on the reasons and evidence discussed here, it is rather clear that long-term use of levodopa in PD patients would accelerate the progression of the disease. In addition, it is also reasoned that the use of COMT inhibitors with preferential peripheral activity would be better as an adjuvant than the centrally-acting COMT inhibitors in the levodopa-based therapy of PD. Because of the neurotoxicity associated with levodopa, it is suggested that noncatechol, centrally-acting dopamine receptor agents could be a better alternative to levodopa for the treatment of PD (particularly for late-stage PD). Lastly, a dietary strategy is proposed to lower the risk of human PD, which includes eating a nutritionally-balanced diet that contains adequate (but not excessive) amounts of fruits, vegetables and whole grains, along with adequate dietary supplementation of SAM, vitamins C, B_6, B_{12}, and folate. More studies are warranted to experimentally test these novel hypotheses. It is believed that the mechanistic understandings developed here may also offer unique insights into the mechanisms of other age-dependent neurodegenerative diseases, such as Huntington's disease.

REFERENCES

[1] Pollanen MS, Dickson DW and Bergeron C: Pathology and biology of the Lewy body. *J Neuropathol Exp Neurol 52:* 183-191, 1993.

[2] Kuzuhara S, Mori H, Izumiyama N, Yoshimura M and Ihara Y: Lewy bodies are ubiquitinated: a light and electron microscopic immunocytochemical study. *Acta Neuropathol (Berl) 75:* 345-353, 1988.

[3] Hoehn MM and Yahr MD: Parkinsonism: onset, progression and mortality. *Neurology 17:* 427-442, 1967.

[4] Tanner CM, Ottman R, Goldman SM, Ellenberg J, Chan P, Mayeux R and Langston JW. Parkinson disease in twins: an etiologic study. *JAMA 281*: 341-346, 1999.

[5] Duvoisin RC and Johnson WG: Hereditary Lewy-body parkinsonism and evidence for a genetic etiology of Parkinson's disease. *Brain Pathol 2*: 309-320, 1992.

[6] Burn DJ, Mark MH, Playford ED, Maraganore DM, Zimmerman TR Jr, Duvoisin RC, Harding AE, Marsden CD and Brooks DJ: Parkinson's disease in twins studied with 18F-dopa and positron emission tomography. *Neurology 42*: 1894-1900, 1992.

[7] Morrish PK, Rakshi JS, Bailey DL, Sawle GV and Brooks DJ: Measuring the rate of progression and estimating the preclinical period of Parkinson's disease with [18F]dopa PET. *J Neurol Neurosurg Psychiatry 64*: 314-319, 1998.

[8] Tang MX, Jacobs D, Stern Y, Marder K, Schofield P, Gurland B, Andrews H and Mayeux R: Risk of Parkinson's disease among first-degree relatives: a community-based study. *Neurology 47*: 155-160, 1996.

[9] Payami H, Larsen K, Bernard S and Nutt J: Increased risk of Parkinson's disease in parents and siblings of patients. *Ann Neurol 36*: 659-661, 1994.

[10] Bennett DA, Beckett LA, Murray AM, Shannon KM, Goetz CG, Pilgrim DM and Evans DA: Prevalence of Parkinsonian signs and associated mortality in a community population of older people. *N Engl J Med 334*: 71-76, 1996.

[11] Piccini P, Morrish PK, Turjanski N, Sawle GV, Burn DJ, Weeks RA, Mark MH, Maraganore DM, Lees AJ and Brooks DJ: Dopaminergic function in familial Parkinson's disease: a clinical and 18F-dopa positron emission tomography study. *Ann Neurol 41*: 222-229, 1997.

[12] Sveinbjörnsdóttir S, Hicks AA, Jónsson T, Pétursson H, Guðmundsson G, Frigge ML, Kong A, Gulcher JR and Stefánsson K: Familial aggregation of Parkinson's disease in Iceland. *N Engl J Med 343*: 1765-1770, 2000.

[13] Nussbaum RL and Ellis CE: Genomic Medicine: Alzheimer's Disease and Parkinson's Disease. *N Engl J Med 348*: 1356-1364, 2003.

[14] Lücking CB, Dürr A, Bonifati V, Vaughan J, De Michele G, Gasser T, Harhangi BS, Meco G, Denèfle P, Wood NW, Agid Y and Brice A: The European consortium on genetic susceptibility in Parkinson's disease and the French Parkinson's disease genetics study group. Association between early-onset Parkinson's disease and mutations in the Parkin Gene. *N Engl J Med 342*: 1560-1567, 2000.

[15] Davis GC, Williams AC, Markey SP, Ebert MH, Caine ED, Reichert CM and Kopin IJ: Chronic Parkinsonism secondary to intravenous injection of meperidine analogues. *Psychiatr Res 1*: 249-254, 1979.

[16] Burns RS, Chiueh CC, Markey SP, Ebert MH, Jacobowitz DM and Kopin IJ: A primate model of parkinsonism: selective destruction of dopaminergic neurons in the pars compacta of the substantia nigra by N-methyl-4-phenyl-1,2,3,6-tetrahydropyridine. *Proc Natl Acad Sci USA 80:* 4546-4550, 1983.

[17] Langston JW, Ballard P, Tetrud JW and Irwin I: Chronic Parkinsonism in humans due to a product of meperidine-analog synthesis. *Science 219*: 979-980, 1983.

[18] Ballard PA, Tetrud JW and Lanston JW: Permnent human parkinsonism due to 1-methyl-4-phenyl-1,2,3,6-tetrahydropyridine (MPTP): seven cases. Neurology 35: 949-956, 1985.

[19] Stern Y: MPTP-induced parkinsonism. *Prog Neurobiol 34*: 107-114, 1990.

[20] Russ H, Mihatsch W, Gerlach M, Riederer P and Przuntek H: Neurochemical and behavioural features induced by chronic low dose treatment with 1-methyl-4-phenyl-1,2,3,6-tetrahydropyridine (MPTP) in the common marmoset: implications for Parkinson's disease*? Neurosci Lett 123*: 115-118, 1991.

[21] Speciale SG: MPTP: insights into parkinsonian neurodegeneration. *Neurotoxicol Teratol 24*: 607-620, 2002.

[22] Jenner P: The contribution of the MPTP-treated primate model to the development of new treatment strategies for Parkinson's disease. *Parkinsonism Relat Disord 9*: 131-137, 2003.

[23] Fahn S and Cohen G: The oxidant stress hypothesis in Parkinson’s disease: evidence supporting it. *Ann Nuerol 32*: 604-812, 1992.

[24] Stokes AH, Hastings TG and Vrana KE: Cytotoxic and genotoxic potential of dopamine. *J Neurosci Res 55*: 659-665, 1999.

[25] Bolton JL, Trush MA, Penning TM, Dryhurst G and Monks TJ: Role of quinones in toxicology. *Chem Res Toxicol 13*: 136-160, 2000.

[26] Cohen G: Oxidative stress, mitochondrial respiration, and Parkinson's disease. *Ann NY Acad Sci 899*: 112-120, 2000.

[27] Cavalieri EL, Rogan EG and Chakravarti D: Initiation of cancer and other diseases by catechol ortho-quinones: a unifying mechanism. *Cell Mol Life Sci 59*: 665-81, 2002.

[28] Cavalieri EL, Li KM, Balu N, Saeed M, Devanesan P, Higginbotham S, Zhao J, Gross ML and Rogan EG: Catechol ortho-quinones: the electrophilic compounds that form depurinating DNA adducts and could initiate cancer and other diseases. *Carcinogenesis 23*: 1071-1077, 2002.

[29] No authors listed: Effects of tocopherol and deprenyl on the progression of disability in early Parkinson's disease. The Parkinson Study Group. *N Engl J Med 328*: 176-183, 1993.

[30] Olanow CW: Oxidation reactions in Parkinson's disease. *Neurology 40(suppl.)*: 32-37, 1990.

[31] Dexter DT, Carter CJ, Wells FR, Javoy-Agid F, Agid Y, Lees A, Jenner P and Marsden CD: Basal lipid peroxidation in substantia nigra is increased in Parkinson's disease. *J Neurochem 52*: 381-389, 1989.

[32] Benzi G, Curti D, Pastoris O, Marzatico F, Villa RF and Dagani F: Sequential damage in mitochondrial complexes by peroxidative stress. *Neurochem Res 16*: 1295-1302, 1991.

[33] Alam ZI, Daniel SE, Lees AJ, Marsden DC, Jenner P and Halliwell B: A generalised increase in protein carbonyls in the brain in Parkinson's but not incidental Lewy body disease. *J Neurochem 69*: 1326-1329, 1997.

[34] Alam ZI, Jenner A, Daniel SE, Lees AJ, Cairns N, Marsden CD, Jenner P and Halliwell B: Oxidative DNA damage in the parkinsonian brain: an apparent selective increase in 8-hydroxyguanine levels in substantia nigra. *J Neurochem 69*: 1196-1203, 1997.

[35] Riederer P, Sofic E, Rausch WD, Schmidt B, Reynolds GP, Jellinger K and Youdim MB: Transition metals, ferritin, glutathione, and ascorbic acid in parkinsonian brains. *J Neurochem 52*: 515-520, 1989.

[36] Sofic E, Lange KW, Jellinger K and Riederer P: Reduced and oxidized glutathione in the substantia nigra of patients with Parkinson's disease. *Neurosci Lett 142*: 128-130, 1992.

[37] Sian J, Dexter DT, Lees AJ, Daniel S, Agid Y, Javoy-Agid F, Jenner P and Marsden CD: Alterations in glutathione levels in Parkinson's disease and other neurodegenerative disorders affecting basal ganglia. *Ann Neurol 36*: 348-355, 1994.

[38] Dexter DT, Sian J, Rose S, Hindmarsh JG, Mann VM, Cooper JM, Wells FR, Daniel SE, Lees AJ, Schapira AH: Indices of oxidative stress and mitochondrial function in individuals with incidental Lewy body disease. *Ann Neurol 35*: 38-44, 1994.

[39] Floor E: Iron as a vulnerability factor in nigrostriatal degeneration in aging and Parkinson's disease. *Cell Mol Biol (Noisy-le-grand) 46*: 709-720, 2000.

[40] Agid Y: Levodopa. Is toxicity a myth? *Neurology 50*: 858-863, 1998.

[41] Fahn S: Is levodopa toxic? *Neurology 47(suppl.):* 184-195, 1996.

[42] Rivett AJ, Eddy B and Roth JA: Contribution of sulfate conjugation, deamination, and O-methylation to metabolism of dopamine and norepinephrine in human brain. *J Neurochem 39:* 1009-1016, 1982.

[43] Kastner A, Anglade P, Bounaix C, Damier P, Javoy-Agid F, Bromet N, Agid Y and Hirsch EC: Immunohistochemical study of catechol-O-methyltransferase in the human mesostriatal system. *Neuroscience 62*: 449-457, 1994.

[44] Werner P, Di Rocco AD, Prikhojan A, Rempel N, Bottiglieri T, Bressman S and Yahr MD: COMT-dependent protection of dopaminergic neurons by methionine, dimethionine and S-adenosylmethionine (SAM) against L-dopa toxicity in vitro. *Brain Res 893*: 278-281, 2001.

[45] Zhu BT: On the mechanism of homocysteine pathophysiology and pathogenesis: A unifying hypothesis. *Histol Histopathol 17*: 1283-1291, 2002.

[46] Zhu BT: Catechol-O-Methyltransferase (COMT)-mediated methylation metabolism of endogenous bioactive catechols and modulation by endobiotics and xenobiotics: importance in pathophysiology and pathogenesis. *Curr Drug Metab 3*: 321-349, 2002.

[47] Durand P, Prost M, Loreau N, Lussier-Cacan S and Blache D: Impaired homocysteine metabolism and atherothrombotic disease. *Lab Invest 81*: 645-672, 2001.

[48] Johnston JM and Kredich NM: Inhibition of methylation by adenosine in adenosine deaminase-inhibited, phytohemagglutinin-stimulated human lymphocytes. *J Immunol 123*: 97-103, 1979.

[49] Kredich NM and Hershfield MS: S-Adenosylhomocysteine toxicity in normal and adenosine kinase-deficient lymphoblasts of human origin. *Proc Natl Acad Sci USA 76*: 2450-2454, 1979.

[50] Kredich NM and Martin DW Jr: Role of S-adenosylhomocysteine in adenosinemediated toxicity in cultured mouse T-lymphoma cells. *Cell 12*: 931-938, 1977.

[51] Helland S and Ueland PM: Reactivation of S-adenosylhomocysteine hydrolase activity in cells exposed to 9-β-D-arabinofuranosyladenine. *Cancer Res 42*: 1130-1136, 1982.

[52] Duerre JA and Briske-Anderson M: Effect of adenosine metabolites on methyltransferase reactions in isolated rat livers. *Biochim Biophys Acta 678*: 275-282, 1981.

[53] Hoffman DR, Marion DW, Cornatzer WE and Duerre JA: S-Adenosylmethionine and S-adenosylhomocystein metabolism in isolated rat liver. Effects of L-methionine, L-homocystein, and adenosine. *J Biol Chem 255*: 10822-10827, 1980.

[54] Schatz RA, Wilens TE and Sellinger OZ: Decreased in vivo protein and phospholipid methylation after in vivo elevation of brain S-adenosyl-homocysteine. *Biochem Biophys Res Commun 98*: 1097-1107, 1981.

[55] Schatz RA, Wilens TE and Sellinger OZ: Decreased transmethylation of biogenic amines after in vivo elevation of brain S-adenosyl-l-homocysteine. *J Neurochem 36*: 1739-1748, 1981.

[56] Ubbink JB, van der Merwe A, Vermaak WJ and Delport R: Hyperhomocysteinemia and the response to vitamin supplementation. *Clin Investig 71*: 993-998, 1993.

[57] Clarke R and Armitage J: Vitamin supplements and cardiovascular risk: review of the randomized trials of homocysteine-lowering vitamin supplements. *Semin Thromb Hermost 26:* 341-348, 2000.

[58] Verhoef P, Stampfer MJ, Buring JE, Gaziano JM, Allen RH, Stabler SP, Reynolds RD, Kok FJ, Hennekens CH and Willett WC: Homocysteine metabolism and risk of myocardial infarction: relation with vitamins B6, B12, and folate. *Am J Epidemiol 143*: 845-859, 1996.

[59] Selhub J, Jacques PF, Wilson PW, Rush D and Rosenberg IH: Vitamin status and intake as primary determinants of homocysteinemia in an elderly population. *J Am Med Assoc 270*: 2693-2698, 1993.

[60] Miller JW: Homocysteine, folate deficiency, and Parkinson's disease. *Nutr Rev 60*: 410-413, 2002.

[61] Mattson MP and Shea TB: Folate and homocysteine metabolism in neural plasticity and neurodegenerative disorders. *Trends Neurosci 26*: 137-146, 2002.

[62] Cotzias GC, Papavasiliou PS and Gellene R: L-Dopa in parkinson's syndrome. *N Engl J Med 280:* 337-345, 1969.

[63] Agid Y, Ahlskog E, Albanese A, Calne D, Chase T, De Yebenes J, Factor S, Fahn S, Gershanik O, Goetz C, Koller W, Kurth M, Lang A, Lees A, Lewitt P, Marsden D, Melamed E, Michel PP, Mizuno Y, Obeso J, Oertel W, Olanow W, Poewe W, Pollak P, Tolosa E, et al.: Levodopa in the treatment of Parkinson's disease: a consensus meeting. *Mov Disord 14*: 911-913, 1999.

[64] Clarke CE and Guttman M: Dopamine agonist monotherapy in Parkinson's disease. *Lancet 360*: 1767-1769, 2002.

[65] Marek K, Jennings D and Seibyl J: Do dopamine agonists or levodopa modify Parkinson's disease progression*? Eur J Neurol. 3(Suppl):* 15-22, 2002.

[66] Männistö PT, Ulmanen I, Lundström K, Taskinen J, Tenhunen J, Tilgmann C and Kaakkola S: Characteristics of catechol O-methyl-transferase (COMT) and properties of selective COMT inhibitors. *Prog Drug Res 39:* 291-350, 1992.

[67] Kuruma I, Bartholini G, Tissot R and Pletscher A: Comparative investigation of inhibitors of extracerebral dopa decarboxylase in man and rats. *J Pharm Pharmacol 24*: 289-294, 1972.

[68] Fahn S: Medical treatment of Parkinson's disease. *J Neurol 245(11 Suppl 3):* P15-24, 1998.

[69] Da Prada M, Keller HH, Pieri L, Kettler R and Haefely WE: The pharmacology of Parkinson's disease: basic aspects and recent advances. *Experientia (Basel) 40*: 1165-1172, 1984.

[70] Rivera-Calimlim L, Tandon D, Anderson F and Joynt R: The clinical picture and plasma levodopa metabolite profile of parkinsonian nonresponders. Treatment with levodopa and decarboxylase inhibitor. *Arch Neurol 34*: 228-232, 1977.

[71] Reilly DK, Rivera-Calimlim L and Van Dyke D: Catechol-O-methyltransferase activity: a determinant of levodopa response. *Clin Pharmacol Ther 28*: 278-286, 1980.

[72] Männisto PT and Kaakkola S: Catechol-O-methyltransferase (COMT): Biochemistry, molecular biology, pharmacology, and clinical efficacy of the new selective COMT inhibitors. *Pharmacol Rev 51*: 593-628, 1999.

[73] Hardie RJ, Malcolm SL, Lees AJ, Stern GM and Allen JG: The pharmacokinetics of intravenous and oral levodopa in patients with Parkinson's disease who exhibit on-off fluctuations. *Br J Clin Pharmacol 22*: 429-436, 1986.

[74] Männistö PT, Kaakkola S, Nissinen E, Lindén I-B and Pohto P: Properties of novel effective and highly selective inhibitors of catechol-O-methyltransferase. *Life Sci 43:* 1465-1471, 1988.

[75] Männistö PT, Tuomainen P and Tuominen RK: Different in vivo properties of three new inhibitors of catechol O-methyltransferase in the rat. *Br J Pharmacol 105*: 569-574, 1992.

[76] Nissinen E, Lindén I-B, Schultz E, Kaakkola S, Männistö PT and Pohto P: Inhibition of catechol-O-methyltransferase activity by two novel disubstituted catechols in the rat. *Eur J Pharmacol 53:* 263-269, 1988.

[77] No authors listed: Entacapone improves motor fluctuations in levodopa-treated Parkinson's disease patients. Parkinson Study Group. *Ann Neurol 42*: 747-755, 1997.

[78] Zhu BT, Ezell EL and Liehr JG: Catechol O methyltransferase catalyzed O methylation of mutagenic flavonoids: Metabolic inactivation as possible reason for their lack of carcinogenicity in vivo. *J Biol Chem 269*: 292 299, 1994.

[79] Zhu BT and Liehr JG: Quercetin increases the severity of estradiol-induced tumorigenesis in hamster kidney. *Toxicol Appl Pharmacol 125*: 149-158, 1994.

[80] Zhu BT and Liehr JG: Inhibition of catechol O-methyltransferase-catalyzed O-methylation of 2- and 4-hydroxyestradiol by quercetin: Possible role in estradiol-induced tumorigenesis. *J Biol Chem 271*: 1357-1363, 1996.

[81] Zhu BT, Patel UK, Cai MX and Conney AH: Metabolic O-methylation of tea polyphenols catalyzed by human placental cytosolic catechol-O-methyltransferase. *Drug Metab Disp 28:* 1024-1030, 2000.

[82] Zhu BT, Patel UK, Cai MX, Lee AJ and Conney AH: Rapid conversion of tea catechins to monomethylated products by rat liver cytosolic catechol-O-methyltransferase. *Xenobiotica 31:* 879-890, 2001.

[83] Nagai M, Conney AH and Zhu BT: Strong inhibitory effects of common tea catechins and bioflavonoids on the O-methylation of catechol estrogens catalyzed by human liver cytosolic catechol-O-methyltransferase. *Drug Metab Disp 32*: 497-504, 2004.

In: Focus on Parkinson's Disease Research
Editor: Marianne J. Willow, pp. 45-63

ISBN 1-59454-924-9
© 2006 Nova Science Publishers, Inc.

Chapter III

The Role of Testosterone and Estrogen in Parkinson's and Other Neurodegenerative Diseases

Tannahill Glen[1], Zighao Huang[1], Gregory Crucian[2] and Michael S. Okun[2*]
[1]Department of Neurology, University of Florida, Jacksonville, FL
[2]Departments of Neurology and Neurosurgery, University of Florida, Movement Disorders Center, Gainesville, FL

Abstract

Parkinson's disease (PD) is a neurodegenerative condition, characterized by motor deficits such as rigidity, tremor, bradykinesia and geit difficulties as well as non-motor symptoms such as cognitive, mood and behavior changes. Recently it has been shown that testosterone may improve refractory non-motor symptoms of PD.This chapter will review the current evidence that estrogen and testosterone may play a role in neurodegenerative diseases such as PD.

Keywords: Testosterone, Strogen, Hormones, Parkinson's, Alzheimer's, Neurodegeration

Introduction

Parkinson's disease (PD) is a neurodegenerative condition, characterized by motor deficits such as rigidity, tremor, bradykinesia and gait difficulties as well as non-motor

* Correspondence concerning this article should be addressed to Dr. Michael S. Okun, Co-Director Movement Disorders Center University of Florida Departments of Neurology, Neurosurgery, and Psychiatry PO Box 100236, Gainesville, FL 32610. 352-392-3491; 352-392-6893 (FAX); Email okun@neurology.ufl.edu.

symptoms such as cognitive, mood and behavior changes. Recently it has been shown that testosterone may improve refractory non-motor symptoms of PD [1,2]. This chapter will review the current evidence that estrogen and testosterone may play a role in neurodegenerative diseases such as PD.

Motor and non-motor symptoms may be explained by dysfunction of one or more of five parallel thalamo-cortical loops, described by Alexander, DeLong and Strick [3]. Each loop originates in a separate area of cerebral cortex. The oculomotor loop originates in the frontal eye fields, and the motor loop in the supplementary motor area. There are also three non-motor or cognitive-behavioral loops that originate in the cingulate, dorsolateral prefrontal and orbitofrontal cortices. According to this model, impairment in PD would relate to the type of information processing mediated by an individual thalamo-cortical loop. Further, the severity of impairment in any domain may be directly proportional to the frontal "load" a specific task may require [4].

Zgaljardic, Borod, Foldi, and Mattis [5], in a comprehensive review of cognitive and behavioral sequelae in PD, elaborated on the three fronto-cortical regions influencing non-motor symptoms of PD. They noted an association between *anterior cingulate* dysfunction and impairment of: 1-attention, 2-response selection/production, 3-initiation and 4-response monitoring. *Dorsolateral prefrontal cortex* was thought to govern: 1-sustained attention, 2-set maintenance, 3-set-shifting and 4-working memory. The dorsolateral prefrontal cortex additionally probably acted as a manager over the three frontal circuits. Orbitofrontal *cortex* was shown to be associated with: 1-disordered social behavior, 2-eating dysfunction, and 3-emotional responses. Perseveration and impairment of strategy formation, inhibition and impulse control have also been noted with orbitofrontal lesions.

Cognitive impairment in patients with PD is characterized by slowed processing, slowed psychomotor speed, loss of mental flexibility, and memory disturbance [6]. Parkinson's disease may also result in the onset of a dementia (PDD) marked by poor spontaneous recall, preserved recognition memory and executive/frontal dysfunction [7]. This pattern of abnormalities has been referred to as a subcortical dementia. However, such a distinction between cortical and subcortical pathology and clinical signs may not be empirically supported [8]. Zakzanis and Freedman [7] suggested that cognitive impairment in PD may be conceptualized as falling along a neuropsychological continuum.

More than half of PD patients exhibit cognitive impairment, while approximately 20% of PD patients have PDD [9]. Estimates of PDD vary widely [8]. This variability may be due to a number of methodological reasons. Criteria for dementia vary, as do assessment measures [8]. Factors such as comorbid diagnoses, age, type of PD (idiopathic versus other parkinsonian syndromes), study location (hospital versus community) and study design (longitudinal versus cross-sectional) all impact and influence current literature [8]. Crucian and Okun [10] published a complete discussion of methodological limitations in the literature on visuospatial ability in PD. These methodological challenges are not specific to visuospatial research and are important to consider when evaluating existing neurocognitive studies on PD. Subject characteristics, comorbidity, symptom laterality, symptom type (e.g., tremor versus bradykinesia/akinesia), fatigue/sleep disturbance, visual acuity, and emotional dysfunction have all been described but are not all accounted for in existing studies of cognitive function in PD.

There may be a relationship between motor and cognitive symptoms in PD [11]. Bradykinesia and rigidity, as well as later age at onset, have been correlated with poor neuropsychological performance [8]. Greater severity of motor impairment was correlated with increased risk for dementia. Tremor was not associated with an increased risk.

Cognitive deficits in PD do not respond well to dopaminergic therapy especially when compared to motor symptoms [4]. Neurotransmitters and non-dopaminergic pathways are therefore likely involved in cognitive dysfunction in PD patients [4,5].

We will review in this chapter the potential role of the sex hormones in cognitive function and PD as well as their role in other neurodegenerative diseases.

Testosterone, Estrogen and Neurobehavior

The preceding review of cognitive, mood and behavior symptoms in PD has suggested that non-motor deficits are common and can be disabling. Therefore, considerable effort has been directed towards determining therapeutic interventions for them. One potentially important consideration is the marked gender differences observed in PD. There is a greater preponderance in males [12,13]. The risk of idiopathic PD in first-degree relatives of PD patients is greater for males than females [14]. Decreased longevity of women with PD has also been noted: women with PD acquire the condition at the same age as men, and have the same progression and duration of disease, but also die at the same age as men. This is in contrast to the longer life expectancy usually noted for women [12]. Women with PD have also been shown to exhibit more levodopa-related dyskinesia compared to men, who exhibit greater severity of parkinsonian motor symptoms [15].

The gender differences in PD are not unique among neurologic disorders. Gender differences have been noted in depression, acquired brain injury, immune disorders, and neurodegenerative conditions [16]. Given that hormonal differences are associated with gender, the role of sex hormones in neurodegenerative disorders will require more study.

Estrogen: Potential Effects on Motor and Non-Motor Features

Most research on the effect of sex hormones on neural functions has focused on estrogen. For example, Gur et al. [17] found gender differences in the effect of aging on brain atrophy, with men showing a significantly greater effect of age (on atrophy). Furthermore, men demonstrated more lateralized atrophy with aging (greater left hemisphere atrophy compared to right), whereas women exhibited more symmetric changes. The authors suggested that female sex hormones may be a protective factor against age-related changes in the brain.

Estrogen has been shown to affect areas of the central nervous system beyond those related to reproduction, such as the hypothalamus [18]. McEwen and Alves, in a thorough review of estrogen's actions on the central nervous system, noted the influence of the ovarian steroid on serotonergic and cholinergic functions, the hippocampus and the spinal cord.

Because of the widespread action of estrogen in the brain, cognition, behavior and mood may also be affected by changes in estrogen levels. Some studies have revealed a relationship between estrogen use after menopause and decreased risk of developing dementia of the Alzheimer's type. Also, research has shown post-menopausal estrogen use in women may delay cognitive deterioration [19, 20]. Estrogen was shown to impact performance on cognitive tests, including memory and spatial measures [21-23]. Estrogen's effect on cognition-related brain activity, using measures of regional cerebral blood flow, has also been demonstrated [24]. The typical pattern of cortical activation noted during completion of the Wisconsin Card Sorting Test was noted to be attenuated and normalized, respectively, by reducing or enhancing the presence of gonadal hormones in young women, even though no changes in task performance were noted clinically.

Other studies have suggested that there are limitations to the measurable effects of estrogen. A study of the effects of short-term estrogen replacement therapy for hypogonadal older men revealed no improvement of cognitive performance [25]. Similarly, studies of the effects of estrogen on depression revealed inconsistent results, with evidence both for and against efficacy of estrogen therapy for depression [25, 26].

Despite those conflicting findings, estrogen treatment was shown, at least in animal studies, to prevent dopamine depletion due to administration of 1-methyl-4-phenyl-1,2,3,6-tetrahydropyridine (MPTP), a substance that has been shown to cause parkinsonism. The neuroprotective effects of estrogen, resulting in reduced dopamine depletion after MPTP administration, were documented in both male and female mice [28, 29]. A neuroprotective effect of estrogen pre-treatment was documented in female mice with methamphetamine-induced nigrostriatal neurotoxicity, but in the same study, post-insult administration of estrogen did not produce the same beneficial effects [30]. Similarly, a neuroprotective effect of estrogen pre-treatment was documented in rats with 6-hydroxydopamine-induced lesions of the nigrostriatal pathway with concomitant protection against loss of motor function [31]. It has also been observed that gender-related differences seem to exist in vulnerability to 6-hydroxydopamine in female rats, where estrogen was a neuroprotective factor, while in male rats, estrogen treatment exacerbated striatal dopamine depletion [32]. The authors cautioned that the beneficial effect of estrogen in females may not generalize to males possibly due to presumed sex differences in the manner in which nigrostriatal dopaminergic neurons respond to estrogen.

Estrogen depletion due to ovariectomy in female rats decreased movement and striatal dopaminergic activity; this effect was reversed in response to twice-weekly (12 weeks) administration [33]. In primates, estrogen deprivation resulted in significant loss of substantia nigra pars compacta dopamine cells. This effect was reversible with estrogen replacement therapy after short-term deprivation (10 days). After longer-term estrogen deprivation, dopamine cell loss was not reversible [34].

The effect of estrogen on PD has been studied in humans. A retrospective study of women with PD by Benedetti et al. [35] revealed that they were significantly more likely to have undergone hysterectomy than normal controls. Although not statistically significant, there was a trend for women with PD to have experienced more episodes of early menopause, and to have used estrogen replacement therapy less frequently after menopause. Additionally, premenstrual increases in PD severity have been reported [36]. However, other studies noted no correlation between estrogen levels and parkinsonism [37]. A retrospective chart review of women with early PD, who were not yet taking L-dopa, revealed greater symptom severity in estrogen naive patients compared to those on estrogen therapy [38].

Inconsistent research findings with estrogen and cognition may be related to methodological limitations, such as lack of randomized trials, and lack of matching subjects on factors such as education and age at onset of symptoms [38]. Also, studies have not clearly defined the role of progesterone or dose-related effects of treatment, or determined that a given compound may act as a pure anti-estrogen [39]. However, estrogen appears to have a modulatory role in PD [40]. Dluzen and Horstink [41] reviewed laboratory and clinical studies of estrogen's functions in the nigrostriatal dopaminergic system, and concluded that they showed evidence for estrogen's role in PD. Saunders-Pullman [40], suggested a neuroprotective role for estrogen in PD, while clinical benefits and the effects of estrogen replacement therapy in PD still remain uncertain. Theories for estrogen's effects have suggested a possible role for neuroprotection by reducing oxidative stress [42], and selective brain receptor targeting (mediating estrogen's effects according to brain region) [39]. Estrogen directly targets dopaminergic neurons, and has been shown to contribute to neuritic branching and dopamine synthesis [43]. The influence of estrogen over gene function has also been examined [44].

We would like to direct the reader to a recent review of estrogen's influence on neurodegenerative disorders by Czlonkowska, Ciesielska and Joniec [16] for a detailed description of the effects of estrogen on neuronal functions, and cellular mechanisms thought to underlie them.

Testosterone and Parkinson's Disease

Testosterone is another sex hormone with significant influence on brain development and function. Prenatal testosterone availability determines gender-related developmental patterns in the brain [45]. For instance, prenatal testosterone availability has been implicated in the asymmetry of the fetal brain, with higher volumes in the male right hemisphere [46]. Testosterone was shown to play a critical role in the developmental organization of the substantia nigra pars reticulata, which has a significant role in motor behavior and contains mostly GABAergic neurons. Although dysfunction of the dopaminergic neurons of the substantia nigra pars compacta has been implicated in PD, the GABAergic system seems to modulate dopaminergic activity [47]. According to McEwen [45], a study of sex differences in brain function should also entail examination of the effects of circulating sex hormones in the adult brain.

The effect of androgen on cortical development persists past the prenatal period. Early administration of testosterone or estradiol was shown to influence neurotransmitter activity (dopamine and serotonin) in newborn rats [48]. Androgen binding and metabolism in rhesus monkey cortex was demonstrated postnatally [49]. Animal studies have revealed a potential increased density of androgen receptors in the dorsolateral and orbitofrontal regions and underlying white matter of adult rhesus monkeys, suggesting contributions to cognitive activity [50]. The prefrontal cortex was also shown to respond to gonadal steroids through adult life. Gonadadectomy in adult male rats preferentially affected the prefrontal cortices compared to sensory and motor cortical regions [51]. Furthermore, changes in both neuroanatomic and behavioral measures were observed in the prefrontal cortex of gonadectomized rats that did not receive testosterone supplementation, compared to rats given the supplement [52]. In humans, sex differences were noted on a measure sensitive to prefrontal cortical functioning: males performed better on the decision-making task, and testosterone levels in young males were negatively correlated with performance [53].

In animal studies, testosterone has been shown to have a role in spatial skills and memory. Performance on an object discrimination reversal task was influenced by gender in rhesus monkeys. Also, lesions of the orbitofrontal area had a differential effect on performance, depending on gender and administration of androgen [54]. Adult male rats with chronic gonadectomy (compared to testosterone-treated rats and controls) exhibited deficits in a spatial maze learning, a task that has been shown to be sensitive to prefrontal cortical dopamine deficiency [55]. Testosterone-related sexual dimorphism in rats has been described [56, 57]. The larger and asymmetrical dentate gyrus granule cell layer in male rat hippocampi was proposed as a possible cause of sex differences in performance on spatial tasks (typically males perform better than females). Also, the authors documented that neonatal testosterone administration resulted in a hippocampus more "male" in appearance. Testosterone administration also improved performance on a spatial maze navigation task. Androgen receptors in the human hippocampus were noted to decline with age, potentially due to age-related neuroendocrine effects and cognitive decline [58].

The potential neuroprotective effect of testosterone was examined by Dluzen [59], who observed the effects of testosterone on MPTP-induced neurotoxicity of the nigrostriatal dopaminergic system in mice. In contrast to studies examining the neuroprotective effects of estrogen, no effect of testosterone on MPTP-induced neurotoxicity was noted, despite evidence of testosterone's effects on nigrostriatal dopamine function. Dluzen suggested that this finding pointed to a possible factor in the gender difference in PD: the greater presence of estrogen in females may have some sort of neuroprotective function in the striatum, and males (who have relatively less estrogen) may thus have greater vulnerability to the disease. A 2001 study by Gao and Dluzen [60] produced similar results. No neuroprotective effect of testosterone on methamphetamine-induced neurotoxicity in male mice was noted. Again, in a study on the effects of estradiol on glutamate-induced neurotoxicity in rat mesencephalic neurons, estradiol adminstration had a neuroprotective effect against stress-induced cell death, while testosterone had no significant effect on cell death in dopaminergic neurons [61]. Likewise, a review of existing studies on testosterone's neuroprotective effects in dementia of the Alzheimer's type found a weak association between testosterone and spatial/memory skills, leading the authors to caution against placing too much emphasis on its effects on cognition, at least in AD, especially given the difficulty comparing results across different studies [62].

However, keeping in mind the interaction between testosterone and the hippocampus, Gouras et al. [63] found that rat neuronal cultures treated with testosterone secreted fewer of the beta-amyloid peptides that compose senile plaques in dementia of the Alzheimer's type. Testosterone replacement in mice was shown to improve age-related decrements in memory and learning; the cognitive impairments were shown to relate to an interaction of aging effects and lower testosterone levels, rather than simply low levels of testosterone [64]. Further evidence for the neuroprotective evidence of androgens was documented in a study of the effect of testosterone on human neuronal cultures [65]. The authors found that testosterone protected against neuronal apoptosis. However, the authors emphasized that testosterone treatment may not be an effective neuroprotectant after androgen receptors have decreased with age, therefore making the timing of intervention potentially critical. Lower testosterone levels were noted in men with dementia of the Alzheimer's type, but it remains unclear whether lower testosterone levels exacerbated or caused the dementing process. The authors advised that future research investigate testosterone levels both prior to and following onset of dementia [66].

Studies on the effects of testosterone deficiency or testosterone replacement in women are extremely limited. Testosterone deficiency in women may result from a number of pathological conditions, such as HIV infection or pituitary disease [67]. Androgen deficiency in women was shown to be associated with menopause, as circulating testosterone levels decreased in the years prior to menopause [68]. Commonly reported symptoms included decreased libido, fatigue and mood problems. Androgen supplementation is currently being studied [69], and some studies have revealed positive effects of testosterone replacement [70]. Dehydroepiandrosterone (DHEA) was investigated as a potential treatment, but studies have revealed inconsistent results in support of its effect on cognition, mood and behavior [71, 72]. Still, there have been some findings that indicate a relationship between testosterone and skills that seem to be influenced by testosterone levels. For example, Gouchie and Kimura [73] demonstrated that women with high salivary testosterone concentrations performed better than women with low levels on measures of spatial/math skills, while no relationship was observed between testosterone levels and performance on measures without sex differences, or measures typically performed better in women. Similarly, a single dose of testosterone in healthy young women was shown to improve object-location memory in only the 3-minute delayed recall portion of the most difficult condition assessed, in which subjects had to reconstruct precise locations, *and* link objects to locations, suggesting a subtle effect of testosterone on spatial memory [74].

There are known consequences of the age-related declines of testosterone in men, described in a thorough review by Tenover [75]. With age, there is a decrease in testosterone production. There are also associated physiological changes such as decreased muscle mass and strength, increased adipose mass, decreased bone mass, decreased libido, erectile dysfunction, and decreased mood. Tenover also noted that these problems, also seen in younger hypogonadal males, may be ameliorated by testosterone replacement. Tenover [76] noted increased lean body mass and weight, and decreased cholesterol, in healthy older males given testosterone. There are some adverse effects of testosterone replacement, however [77]. It was observed [76] that there may be an increase in serum PSA levels after receiving testosterone, consistent with research showing the therapy may be contraindicated when there is a diagnosis of prostate or breast cancer. Testosterone therapy may also increase the risk of fluid retention, sleep apnea (or worsen it), gynecomastia, increased red blood cell mass, prostate disease, and cardiovascular disease [75]. However, it should be noted that testosterone levels in healthy men are quite variable, and not all men will become hypogonadal or exhibit testosterone deficiency with age [78].

Age-related testosterone decline in men has been shown to have an effect on mood, but findings have been inconsistent. Testosterone levels in men were not associated with depression [79]. Another study examined depression, anxiety and quality of life in older men. Testosterone levels were not significantly different for men with high scores on a measure of depressed mood compared to men with lower scores on the same test. Still, a negative correlation was observed between severity of depression and testosterone levels [80]. The authors suggested that age-related testosterone declines may be associated with milder depressive symptoms, rather than clinical depression. In a separate review, it was proposed that psychological symptoms commonly associated with age-related hypogonadism were not specific to the condition, and likely related to a number of contributing factors [81]. Siedman [82] proposed a similar explanation for the symptoms of age-associated testosterone deficiency. This was consistent with another study in which mild mood symptoms were observed in healthy older men, but those symptoms were not correlated with testosterone levels [83]. However, in a large study of older men, higher scores on measures of depression were associated with lower levels of bioavailable testosterone, and levels of testosterone were significantly lower in depressed men compared to men without depression [84].

Testosterone levels in men with major depression have also been examined. Testosterone levels in depressed males and normal males were compared in one study. They were negatively correlated with age, but not severity of depression [85]. Davies, Harris, Thomas, Cook, Read, & Riad-Fahmy [86] found no significant differences in salivary testosterone levels in age-matched controls. However, men with depression who underwent a standard dexamethasone suppression test exhibited a significant negative correlation between pre-dexamethasone levels and scores on measures of depression and anxiety. A small study examined the effect of testosterone replacement on men with low levels of testosterone and depression that did not respond to treatment with a selective serotonin reuptake inhibitor [87]. Interestingly, testosterone therapy was associated with rapid and significant reduction of depressive symptoms and also increased life satisfaction ratings. Furthermore, three of four men who underwent placebo discontinuation of therapy experienced relapse of depression. However, the study's design, with no placebo control, small *n*, and continuation of the SSRI during the course of therapy, made the results uncertain. A larger study of mood symptoms in hypogonadal men demonstrated the positive effect of testosterone replacement therapy on mood [88]. The authors documented an increase in positive mood, and a decrease in negative mood in treated hypogonadal men. Also, positive mood was associated with higher testosterone levels, while negative mood was associated with lower testosterone levels. Because improvement in positive mood scores was also correlated with increased sexual motivation scores, and a decrease in negative mood was associated with improvement in sexual performance, the authors proposed that mood changes may have related to improvement in sexual function. The effects of supraphysiologic levels of testosterone on mood and sexuality in normal men have also been studied [89]. Sexual interest was stimulated by testosterone administration, but no alteration of mood was noted. Wang et al. [88] suggested this may have reflected a threshold effect of testosterone levels: once an optimal level is reached, no further changes in mood/behavior are noted.

Many studies have shown a negative effect of testosterone deficiency on cognition in males. For instance, Barrett-Connor, Goodman-Gruen and Patay [90] studied levels of estradiol and also bioavailable testosterone in older men. Bioavailable testosterone refers to plasma testosterone (freely circulating or albumin-bound) that are available to the brain, and not bound to sex-hormone binding globulin [91]. Barrett-Connor et al. found that older men with higher levels of bioavailable testosterone (BT) performed better on measures of memory, while men with higher levels of estradiol performed more poorly on measures of memory and mental status. Decreases in BT correlated with age-related physical decrements and also verbal and visual learning decrements in healthy males [92]. A subset of males with hypogonadotropic hypogonadism was noted to exhibit mirror movements and spatial attentional abnormalities, and provided supporting evidence for a relationship between testosterone levels and spatial skills [93]. Similarly, another study measured free testosterone and cognitive performance in older men [79]. The authors found that hypogonadal men performed significantly worse on measures of spatial cognition compared to men with more optimal testosterone levels. Men classified as hypogonadal tended to show faster rates of decline on a visual memory test. Further, higher testosterone concentrations, even when levels were still in the normal range, were associated with better performance on spatial cognition tasks and also verbal memory tasks.

Other studies have assessed the effects of testosterone supplementation or replacement, as opposed to simply testosterone levels. Twelve months of testosterone replacement therapy in older hypogonadal men was not associated with changes in verbal or visual memory. However, significant findings may have been difficult to detect due to small sample size and high drop-out rate [94]. A short course of testosterone treatment for older men with low testosterone levels and mild-to-moderate cognitive impairment did not result in changes in behavior, physical functions or cognition [95]. However, the authors suggested the results were evidence of tolerability of the treatment for older men with cognitive impairment, adding that significant changes in cognition may have been missed due to several reasons, including test insensitivity and administration of testosterone following, rather than prior to, cognitive decline. Janowsky, Chavez and Orwoll [96] studied the effects of sex hormones on age-related working memory decrements in older women and men. They found that testosterone supplementation improved working memory in older men, but estrogen supplement did not enhance working memory in older women. Kenny, Bellantonio, Gruman, Acosta, and Prestwood [97] examined the effect on cognition of one year of transdermal testosterone replacement for older men with low testosterone levels. They found that testosterone replacement was associated with significant improvement from baseline on a measure of mental flexibility, and 12-month testosterone levels were associated with changes in the test scores. Cherrier et al. [98] examined the relationship between testosterone administration and visual and verbal memory in healthy older men. Improvement in visual memory, as well as spatial skills, was observed following testosterone administration. Intriguingly, improvement in verbal memory was also demonstrated. This finding was thought to perhaps reflect increased levels of estradiol in response to the testosterone treatment.

Verbal fluency in hypogonadal males improved to normal levels following administration of testosterone [99]. Performance on most other measures of cognitive ability, including spatial skills, was unaffected by testosterone treatment. The authors noted the results may have reflected the effect of testosterone on cortical areas where androgen receptors were located. Alternately, they suggested the possibility that testosterone administration may have increased estradiol levels, thus enhancing verbal fluency. Kenny et al. [97] found increases in estrone, but not estradiol, after testosterone replacement. It is now believed that testosterone has both a direct and indirect (through aromatization of testosterone to estradiol) on the brain [77].

Van Goozen, Cohen-Kettenis, Gooren, Frijda, and Van de Pol [100] examined the effects of cross-sex hormone treatment in female-to-male and also male-to-female transsexuals. Androgen treatment for females resulted in increased aggression, sexual arousal and spatial skill performance, while verbal fluency performance declined. Androgen deprivation in males resulted in the opposite pattern: verbal fluency improved, while aggression, sexual arousal and spatial skills declined. Another study investigated the hypothesis that testosterone replacement in older males would enhance spatial skills and compromise verbal skills [101]. No effect of testosterone was noted on spatial tasks and most verbal tasks. However, 5 days post-treatment, the placebo group exhibited a practice effect on a verbal fluency task that the testosterone group did not exhibit; thus verbal fluency was significantly worse in the testosterone group. The authors suggested that the study's design (examination of cognitive performance after a single injection of testosterone) may have diminished chances of measurable change after treatment.

One study examined the longer-term effects of androgen deprivation on cognition [102]. Androgen deprivation is a common treatment option in prostate cancer. At 12 months post-anti-androgen therapy, patients with prostate cancer exhibited no cognitive impairment compared to pre-treatment baseline performance, despite increased physical complaints. Also, no changes in social or emotional functioning were noted. Thus, despite evidence suggesting cognitive decline may result from lower testosterone levels, this particular intervention may not result in long-term cognitive sequelae. This finding however is questionable and will need replication. However, androgen deprivation therapy was associated with cognitive decline in one case study of an 80 year-old male with dementia of the Alzheimer's type and prostate cancer [103].

The same methodological considerations that contribute to discrepant findings in studies in PD also apply in studies on the effects of testosterone. Sternbach [78] noted that discrepant findings could have reflected differences in patient age, method of measuring testosterone, or factors that may affect testosterone levels such as cortisol levels, weight loss or medication use. Other concerns included the wide array of cognitive measures used, small sample sizes, and the variety of study designs making comparison of results difficult.

Testosterone and Parkinson's Disease: (A Potential Treatment)

There are few empirical studies on the effects of testosterone in PD. Okun, McDonald, and DeLong [1] described improvements with testosterone treatment of refractory nonmotor symptoms in male PD patients. The authors noted that nonmotor symptoms, including problems with cognition, mood and sexual functioning, have received less attention in research on PD treatment. These symptoms are sometimes attributable to identifiable comorbid conditions in PD, such as depression, sleep disorders and hypothyroidism. Okun et al. described another common comorbid condition in PD, testosterone deficiency. The symptoms of testosterone deficiency, as described in the previous section, are quite similar to the nonmotor symptoms in PD, and may respond positively to testosterone replacement therapy. Five male PD patients with refractory nonmotor symptoms received testosterone replacement therapy. All 5 patients reported significant improvement in previously refractory symptoms, such as mood, mobility, energy, libido and strength. Of course, the small sample size and lack of placebo control limited interpretation of results. The authors also examined data from a PD registry, and found that 35% of men with PD exhibited low testosterone levels. This was higher than the 20%-25% of healthy males older than 60 who exhibit testosterone deficiency [104]. They also noted a significant relationship between increasing age and testosterone deficiency, similar to the normal older male population.

Okun et al. [2] then designed an open-label pilot study to examine testosterone replacement in PD. Ten male non-demented PD patients with testosterone deficiency were administered a single daily dose of testosterone replacement gel for one month. Outcome measures included testosterone deficiency symptoms, PD symptoms (motor and nonmotor), dyskinesia, quality of life, sleepiness, mood and neuropsychological functions (verbal fluency, and attention/concentration). These were administered at baseline, 1 month, and 3 months post-treatment. Results indicated increases in testosterone levels and improvement in testosterone deficiency symptoms, such as energy level, libido and enjoyment. PD-related motor fluctuations showed improvement at 1 month post-treatment, but not at 3 months. PD-related intellectual function as measured by the Unified Parkinson's Disease Rating Scale (UPDRS) showed improvement at 3 months post-treatment. Verbal fluency improved at 3 months follow-up. Anxiety improved at one month post-treatment but this improvement was not sustained at follow-up. Because only 4 out of 10 patients exhibited a doubling of testosterone levels, the authors addressed several issues. First, inability to increase testosterone levels in several participants may have masked significant findings in the pilot study. Second, there was the question of whether higher dose of testosterone would have resulted in greater improvement in outcome measures. Finally, the possible role of the placebo effect on results was important to consider. There were other methodological considerations in this study. For example, treatment and follow-up intervals may have been abbreviated, and the method of testosterone administration (gel versus intramuscular injection) may have been less than optimal for the study design.

The most recent examination of testosterone in PD is a study by Okun, DeLong, Hanfelt, Gearing, & Levey [105]. The authors studied 68 male PD patients and 50 male patients with dementia of the Alzheimer's type. Plasma testosterone levels were obtained, and comprehensive neuropsychological assessment was performed. Testosterone levels in PD and AD were compared, and the relationship between neuropsychological performance and testosterone levels was analyzed. The authors found no significant differences in testosterone levels between PD and AD groups. Age-related decline in testosterone levels was observed, but the rate of decline did not differ between groups. However, rate of decline in the PD/AD groups was greater than the rate of decline in a community sample of aging males. In terms of performance on cognitive measures, only performance on time needed for completion of the Trailmaking Test B (a measure of mental flexibility) showed a significant difference. PD patients with lower testosterone levels performed more poorly on the test when adjusting for age and education.

Directions for Future Research

With regard to the impact of sex hormones in neurodegenerative disorders such as PD, there are two issues. First, it remains unclear whether testosterone exerts a neuroprotective effect on the nigrostriatal dopmainergic system. The second issue concerns the proposed modulatory effect of testosterone on cognition, mood and behavior. Evidence from existing studies has been conflicting, hampered by small sample sizes, lack of placebo and normal controls, use of varied measures, different study designs and methodology, varied patient groups, and nonstandardized diagnostic decision-making, such as discrepancies in defining PD-related dementia or even testosterone deficiency. However, a significant body of research exists suggesting a relationship between testosterone and non-motor symptoms of PD. Future research must identify the individual domains that may be affected by testosterone and estrogen, and move toward well-designed studies in the PD population. Studies such as these will help elucidate the role of sex steroids in neurodegerative diseases such as PD. Given the inherent difficulty in comparing results across studies, future research that addresses the methodological issues noted above may provide more definitive evidence, and in turn provide direction for more comprehensive treatment of motor and non-motor symptoms in PD, as well as identify factors contributing to the sex difference.

Acknowledgment

The authors would like to acknowledge Cody Westmoreland, Research Assistant, for her help in preparation of this manuscript. The authors would also like to thank the Michael J. Fox Foundation for their support of the study of Testosterone and Parkinson's Disease (Principle Investigators- Okun, Crucian), and the National Parkinson Foundation.

References

[1] Okun MS, McDonald WM, Delong MR. Refractory nonmotor symptoms in male patients with Parkinson disease due to testosterone deficiency: a common unrecognized comorbidity. *Arch Neurol.* 2002;59: 807-811.

[2] Okun MS, Walter BL, McDonald WM, Tenover JL, Green J, Juncos JL, Delong MR. Beneficial effects of testosterone replacement for the nonmotor symptoms of Parkinson disease. *Arch Neurol.* 2002;59:1750-1753.

[3] Alexander GE, Delong MR, Strick PL. Parallel organization of functionally segregated circuits linking basal ganglia and cortex. *Annu Rev Neurosci.* 1986;9:357-381.

[4] Taylor AE, Saint-Cyr JA. The neuropsychology of Parkinson's disease. *Brain Cogn.* 1995;28: 281-296.

[5] Zgaljardic DJ, Borod JC, Foldi NS, Mattis P. A review of the cognitive and behavioral sequelae of Parkinson's disease: relationship to frontostriatal circuitry. *Cogn Behav Neurol.* 2003;16:193-210.

[6] Lezak MD. (1995). Neuropsychological Assessment (3rd ed). New York: Oxford University Press.

[7] Zakzanis KK, Freedman M. A neuropsychological comparison of demented and nondemented patients with Parkinson's disease. *Appl Neuropsychol.* 1999;6:129-146.

[8] Pahwa R, Paolo A, Tröster A, Koller W. Cognitive impairment in Parkinson's disease. *Eur J Neurol.* 1998;5:431-441.

[9] Lee C, Grossman M, Morris J, Stern MB, Hurtig HI. Attentional resource and processing speed limitations during sentence processing in Parkinson's disease. *Brain Lang.* 2003;85:347-356.

[10] Crucian GP, Okun MS. Visual-spatial ability in Parkinson's disease. *Front Biosci.* 2003;8: s992-7.

[11] Marder K, Tang MX, Cote L, Stern Y, Mayeux R. The frequency and associated risk factors for dementia in patients with Parkinson's disease. *Arch Neurol.* 1995;52:695-701.

[12] Diamond SG, Markham CH, Hoehn MM, McDowell FH, Muenter MD. An examination of male-female differences in progression and mortality of Parkinson's disease. *Neurology.* 1990;40:763-766.

[13] Mayeux R, Denaro J, Hemenegildo N, Marder K, Tang MX, Cote LJ, Stern Y. A population-based investigation of Parkinson's disease with and without dementia: relationship to age and gender. *Arch Neurol.* 1992;49:492-497.

[14] Marder K, Tang MX, Mejia H, Alfaro B, Cote L, Louis E, Groves J, Mayeux R. Risk of Parkinson's disease among first-degree relatives: a community-based study. *Neurology.* 1996;47:155-160.

[15] Lyons KE, Hubble JP, Tröster AI, Pahwa R, Koller WC. Gender differences in Parkinson's disease. *Clin Neuropharmacol.* 1998;21:118-121.

[16] Czlonkowska A, Ciesielska A, Joniec I. Influence of estrogens on neurodegenerative processes. *Med Sci Monit.* 2003;9:RA247-256.

[17] Gur RC, Mozley PD, Resnick SM, Gottlieb GL, Kohn M, Zimmerman R, Herman G, Atlas S, Grossman R, Berretta D, et al. Gender differences in age effect on brain atrophy measured by magnetic resonance imaging. *Proc Natl Acad Sci USA.* 1991;88:2845-2849.

[18] McEwen BS, Alves SE. Estrogen actions in the central nervous system. *Endocr Rev.* 1999; 20:279-307.

[19] Costa MM, Reus VI, Wolkowitz OM, Manfredi F, Lieberman M. Estrogen replacement therapy and cognitive decline in memory-impaired post-menopausal women. *Biol Psychiatry.* 1999; 46:182-188.

[20] Tang MX, Jacobs D, Stern Y, Marder K, Schofield P, Gurland B, Andrews H, Mayeux R. Effect of oestrogen during menopause on risk and age at onset of Alzheimer's disease. *Lancet.* 1996; 348:429-432.

[21] Shilling V, Jenkins V, Fallowfield L, Howell T. The effects of hormone therapy on cognition in breast cancer. *J Steroid Biochem Mol Biol.* 2003; 86:405-412.

[22] Bimonte-Nelson HA, Singleton RS, Hunter CL, Price KL, Moore AB, Granholm AC. Ovarian hormones and cognition in the aged female rat: I. Long term, but not short-term, ovariectomy enhances spatial performance. *Behav Neurosci.* 2003;117:1395-1406.

[23] Sherwin BB. Estrogen effects on cognition in menopausal women. *Neurology.* 1997;48: S21-26.

[24] Berman KF, Schmidt PJ, Rubinow DR, Danaceau MA, Van Horn JD, Esposito G, Ostrem JL, Weinberger DR. Modulation of cognition-specific cortical activity by gonadal steroids: a positron-emission tomography study in women. *Proc Natl Acad Sci USA.* 1997;94: 8836-8841.

[25] Taxel P, Stevens MC, Trahiotis M, Zimmerman J, Kaplan RF. The effect of short-term estradiol therapy on cognitive function in older men receiving hormonal suppression therapy for prostate cancer. *J Am Geriatr Soc.* 2004;52:269-273.

[26] Morrison MF, Kallan MJ, Ten Have T, Katz I, Tweedy K, Battistini M. Lack of efficacy of estradiol for depression in postmenopausal women: a randomized, controlled trial. *Biol Psychiatry.* 2004;55:406-412.

[27] Miller KJ. The other side of estrogen replacement therapy: outcome study results of mood improvement in estrogen users and nonusers. *Curr Psychiatry.* 2003;5:439-444.

[28] Dluzen DE, McDermott JL, Liu B. Estrogen as a neuroprotectant against MPTP-induced neurotoxicity in C57/B1 mice. *Neurotoxicol Teratol.* 1996;18:603-606.

[29] Miller DB, Ali SF, O'Callaghan JP, Laws SC. The impact of gender and estrogen on striatal dopaminergic neurotoxicity. *Ann N Y Acad Sci.* 1998;844:153-165.

[30] Gajjar TM, Anderson LI, Dluzen DE. Acute effects of estrogen upon methamphetamine induced neurotoxicity of the nigrostriatal dopaminergic system. *J Neural Transm.* 2003;110:1215-1224.

[31] Quesada A, Micevych PE. Estrogen interacts with the IGF-1 system to protect nigrostriata dopamine and maintain motoric behavior after 6-hydroxdopamine lesions. *J Neurosci Res.* 2004;75:107-116.

[32] Murray HE, Pillai AV, McArthur SR, Razvi N, Datla KP, Dexter DT, Gillies GE. Dose- and sex-dependent effects of the neurotoxin 6-hydroxydopamine on the nigrostriatal dopaminergic pathway of adult rats: differential actions of estrogen in males and females. *Neuroscience.* 2003;116:213-222.

[33] Ohtani H, Nomoto M, Douchi T. Chronic estrogen treatment replaces striatal dopaminergic function in ovariectomized rats. *Brain Res.* 2001;900:163-168.

[34] Leranth C, Roth RH, Elswoth JD, Naftolin F, Horvath TL, Redmond DE Jr. Estrogen is essential for maintaining nigrostriatal dopamine neurons in primates: implications for Parkinson's disease and memory. *J Neurosci.* 2000;20:8604-8609.

[35] Benedetti MD, Maraganore DM, Bower JH, McDonnell SK, Peterson BJ, Ahlskog JE, Schaid DJ, Rocca WA. Hysterectomy, menopause, and estrogen use preceding Parkinson's disease: an exploratory case-control study. *Mov Disord.* 2001;16:830-837.

[36] Quinn NP, Marsden CD. Menstrual-related fluctuations in Parkinson's disease. *Mov Disord.* 1986;1:85-87. Abstract.

[37] Kompoliti K, Comella CL, Jaglin JA, Leurgans S, Raman R, Goetz CG. Menstrual-related changes in motoric function in women with Parkinson's disease. *Neurology*. 2000;55:1572-1575.

[38] Saunders-Pullman R, Gordon-Elliot J, Parides M, Fahn S, Saunders HR, Bressman S. The effect of estrogen replacement on early Parkinson's disease. *Neurology*. 1999;52:1417-1421.

[39] Cyr M, Calon F, Morissette M, Di Paolo T. Estrogenic modulation of brain activity: implications for schizophrenia and Parkinson's disease. *J Psychiatry Neurosci*. 2002;27:12-27.

[40] Saunders-Pullman R. Estrogens and Parkinson disease: neuroprotective, symptomatic, neither, or both? *Endocrine*. 2003;21:81-87.

[41] Dluzen D, Horstink M. Estrogen as neuroprotectant of nigrostriatal dopaminergic system: laboratory and clinical studies. *Endocrine*. 2003;21:67-75.

[42] Behl C, Moosmann B, Manthey D, Heck S. The female sex hormone oestrogen as neuroprotectant: activities at various levels. *Novartis Found Symp*. 2000;230:221-234.

[43] Kuppers E, Ivanova T, Karolczak M, Beyer C. Estrogen: a multifunctional messenger to nigrostriatal dopaminergic neurons. *J Neurocytol*. 2000;29:375-385.

[44] Huber JC, Schneeberger C, Tempfer CB. Genetic modeling of estrogen metabolism as a risk factor of hormone-dependent disorders. *Maturitas*. 2002;41:*S55-64*.

[45] McEwen BS. Permanence of brain sex differences and structural plasticity of the adult brain. *Proc Natl Acad Sci USA*. 1999;96:7128-7130.

[46] de Lacoste MC, Horvath DS, Woodward DJ. Possible sex differences in the developing human fetal brain. *J Clin Exp Neuropsychol*. 1991;13:831-846.

[47] Velísková J, Moshé SL. Sexual dimorphism and developmental regulation of substantia nigra function. *Ann Neurol*. 2001;50:596-601.

[48] Dominguez R, Cruz-Morales SE, Carvalho MC, Xavier M, Brandao ML. Effect of steroid injection to newborn rats on serotonin activity in frontal cortex and raphe. *Neuroreport*. 2003;14:597-599.

[49] Clark AS, MacLusky NJ, Goldman-Rakic PS. Androgen binding and metabolism in the cerebral cortex of the developing rhesus monkey. *Endocrinology*. 1988;123:932-940.

[50] Finley SK, Kritzer MF. Immunoreactivity for intracellular androgen receptors in identified subpopulations of neurons, astrocytes and oligodendrocytes in primate prefrontal cortex. *J Neurobiol*. 1999;40:446-457.

[51] Kritzer MF, Adler A, Marotta J, Smirlis T. Regionally selective effects of gonadectomy on cortical catecholamine innervation in adult male rats are most disruptive to afferents in prefrontal cortex. *Cereb Cortex*. 1999;9:507-518.

[52] Adler A, Vescovo P, Robinson JK, Kritzer MF. Gonadectomy in adult life increases tyrosine hydroxylase immunoreactivity in the prefrontal cortex and decreases open field activity in male rats. *Neuroscience*. 1999;89:939-954.

[53] Reavis R, Overman WH. Adult sex differences on a decision-making task previously shown to depend on the orbital prefrontal cortex. *Behav Neurosci*. 2001;115:196-206.

[54] Clark AS, Goldman-Rakic PS. Gonadal hormones influence the emergence of cortical function in nonhuman primates. *Behav Neurosci*. 1989;103:1287-1295.

[55] Kritzer MF, McLaughlin PJ, Smirlis T, Robinson JK. Gonadectomy impairs T-maze acquisition in adult male rats. *Horm Behav*. 2001;39:167-174.

[56] Roof RL, Havens MD. Testosterone improves maze performance and induces development of a male hippocampus in females. *Brain Res*. 1992;572:310-313.

[57] Roof RL. The dentate gyrus is sexually dimorphic in prepubescent rats: testosterone plays a significant role. *Brain Res*. 1993;610:148-151.

[58] Tohgi H, Utsugisawa K, Yamagata M, Yoshimura M. Effects of age on messenger RNA expression of glucocorticoid, thyroid hormone, androgen, and estrogen receptors in postmortem human hippocampus. *Brain Res*. 1995;700:245-253.

[59] Dluzen DE. Effects of testosterone upon MPTP-induced neurotoxicity of the nigrostriatal dopaminergic system of C57/B1 mice. *Brain Res*. 1996;715:113-118.

[60] Gao X, Dluzen DE. The effect of testosterone upon methamphetamine neurotoxicity of the nigrostriatal dopaminergic system. *Brain Res*. 2001;892:63-69.

[61] Sawada H, Ibi M, Kihara T, Urushitani M, Akaike A, Shimohama S. Estradiol protects mesencephalic dopaminergic neurons from oxidative stress-induced neuronal death. *J Neurosci Res*. 1998;54:707-719.

[62] Almeida OP, Flicker L. Testosterone and dementia: too much ado about too little data. *J Br Menopause Soc*. 2003;9:107-110.

[63] Gouras GK, Xu H, Gross RS, Greenfield JP, Hai B, Wang R, Greengard P. Testosterone reduces neuronal secretion of Alzheimer's ß–amyloid peptides. *Proc Nat'l Acad Sci USA*. 2000;97:1202-1205.

[64] Flood JF, Farr SA, Kaiser FE, La Regina M, Morley JE. Age-related decrease of plasma testosterone in SAMP8 mice: replacement improves age-related impairment of learning and memory. *Physiol Behav*. 1995;57:669-673.

[65] Hammond J, Le Q, Goodyer C, Gelfand M, Trifiro M, LeBlanc A. Testosterone-mediated neuroprotection through the androgen receptor in human primary neurons. *J Neurochem*. 2001;77:1319-1326.

[66] Hogervorst E, Williams J, Budge M, Barnetson L, Combrinck M, Smith AD. Serum total testosterone is lower in men with Alzheimer's disease. *Neuroendocrinol Lett*. 2001;22:163-168.

[67] Mazer NA. Testosterone deficiency in women: etiologies, diagnosis, and emerging treatments. *Int J Fertil Womens Med*. 2002;47:77-86.

[68] Burd ID, Bachmann GA. Androgen replacement in menopause. *Curr Womens Health Rep*. 2001;1:202-205.

[69] Davison SL, Davis SR. Androgens in women. *J Steroid Biochem Mol Biol*. 2003;85:363-366.

[70] Davis SR, Tran J. Testosterone influences libido and well being in women. *Trends Endocrinol Metab*. 2001;12:33-37.

[71] Strous RD, Maayan R, Lapidus R, Stryjer R, Lustig M, Kotler M, Weizman A. Dehydroepiandrosterone augmentation in the management of negative, depressive, and anxiety symptoms in schizophrenia. *Arch Gen Psychiatry*. 2003;60:133-141.

[72] Wolkowitz OM, Kramer JH, Reus VI, Costa MM, Yaffe K, Walton P, Raskind M, Peskind E, Newhouse P, Sack D, De Souza E, Sadowsky C, Roberts E. DHEA

treatment of Alzheimer's disease: a randomized, double-blind, placebo-controlled study. *Neurology*. 2003;60:1071-1076.

[73] Gouchie C, Kimura D. The relationship between testosterone levels and cognitive ability patterns. *Psychoneuroendocrinology*. 1991;16:323-334.

[74] Postma A, Meyer G, Tuiten A, van Honk J, Kessels RPC, Thijssen J. Effects of testosterone administration on selective aspects of object-location memory in healthy young women. *Psychoneuroendocrinology*. 2000;25:563-575.

[75] Tenover JL. Testosterone replacement therapy in older adult men. *Int J Androl*. 1999;22:300-306.

[76] Tenover JS. Effects of testosterone supplementation in the aging male. *J Clin Endocrinol Metab*. 1992;75:1092-1098.

[77] Tan RS, Culberson JW. An integrative review on current evidence of testosterone replacement therapy for the andropause. *Maturitas*. 2002;45:15-27.

[78] Sternbach H. Age-associated testosterone decline in men: clinical issues for psychiatry. *Am J Psychiatry*. 1998;155:1310-1318.

[79] Moffat SD, Zonderman AB, Metter EJ, Blackman MR, Harman SM, Resnick SM. Longitudinal assessment of serum free testosterone concentration predicts memory performance and cognitive status in elderly men. *J Clin Endocrinol Metab*. 2002;87:5001-5007.

[80] Delhez M, Hansenne M, Legros JJ. Andropause and psychopathology: minor symptoms rather than pathological ones. *Psychoneuroendocrinology*. 2003;28:863-874.

[81] Delhez M, Hansenne M, Legros JJ. Testosterone and depression in men aged over 50 years: andropause and psychopathology: minimal systemic work-up. *Ann Endocrinol*. 2003;64:162-169.

[82] Seidman SN. Testosterone deficiency and mood in aging men: pathogenic and therapeutic interactions. *World J Biol Psychiatry*. 2003;4:14-20.

[83] T'Sjoen G, Goemaere S, De Meyere M, Kaufman JM. Perception of males' aging symptoms, health and well-being in elderly community-dwelling men is not related to circulating androgen levels. *Psychoneuroendocrinology*. 2004;29:201-214.

[84] Barrett-Conner E, Von Muhlen DG, Kritz-Silverstein D. Bioavailable testosterone and depressed mood in older men: the Rancho Bernardo study. *J Clin Endocrinol Metab*. 1999;84:573-577.

[85] Levitt AJ, Joffe RT. Total and free testosterone in depressed men. *Acta Psychiatr Scand*. 1988;77:346-348. Abstract.

[86] Davies RH, Harris B, Thomas DR, Cook N, Read G, Riad-Fahmy D. Salivary testosterone levels and major depressive illness in men. *Br J Psychiatry*. 1992;161:629-632.

[87] Seidman SN, Rabkin JG. Testosterone replacement therapy for hypogonadal men with SSRI-refractory depression. *J Affect Disord*. 1998;48:157-161.

[88] Wang C, Alexander G, Berman N, Salehian B, Davidson T, McDonald V, Steiner B, Hull L, Callegari C, Swerdloff RS. Testosterone replacement therapy improves mood in hypogonadal men: a clinical research center study. *J Clin Endocrinol Metab*. 1996;81:3578-3583.

[89] Anderson RA, Bancroft J, Wu FCW. The effects of exogenous testosterone on sexuality and mood of normal men. *J Clin Endocrinol Metab*. 1992;75:1503-1507.

[90] Barrett-Conner E, Goodman-Gruen D, Patay B. Endogenous sex hormones and cognitive function in older men. *J Clin Endocrinol Metab*. 1999;84:3681-3685.

[91] Pardridge WM, Landaw EM. Testosterone transport in brain: primary role of plasma protein bound hormone. *Am J Physiol*. 1985;249:E534-542.

[92] Morley JE, Kaiser F, Raum WJ, Perry HM III, Flood JF, Jensen J, Silver AJ, Roberts E. Potentially predictive and manipulable blood serum correlates of aging in the healthy human male: progressive decreases in bioavailable testosterone, dehydroepiandrosterone sulfate, and the ratio of insulin-like growth factor 1 to growth hormone. *Proc Natl Acad Sci USA*. 1997;94:7537-7542.

[93] Kertzman C, Robinson DL, Sherins RJ, Schwankhaus JD, McClurkin JW. Abnormalities in visual spatial attention in men with mirror movements associated with isolated hypogonadotropic hypogonadism. *Neurology*. 1990;40:1057-1063.

[94] Sih R, Morley JE, Kaiser FE, Perry HM III, Patrick P, Ross C. Testosterone replacement in older hypogonadal men: a 12-month randomized controlled trial. *J Clin Endocrinol Metab*. 1997;82:1661-1667.

[95] Kenny AM, Fabregas G, Song C, Biskup B, Bellantonio S. Effects of testosterone on behavior, depression, and cognitive function in older men with mild cognitive loss. *J Gerontol Med Sci*. 2004;59A:75-78.

[96] Janowsky JS, Chavez B, Orwoll E. Sex steroids modify working memory. *J Cogn Neurosci*. 2000;12:407-414.

[97] Kenny AM, Bellantonio S, Gruman CA, Acosta RD, Prestwood KM. Effects of transdermal testosterone on cognitive function and health perception in older men with low bioavailable testosterone levels. *J Gerontol A Biol Aci Med Sci*. 2002;57:M321-325.

[98] Cherrier MM, Asthana S, Plymate S, Baker L, Matsumoto AM, Peskind E, Raskind MA, Brodkin K, Bremner W, Petrova A, LaTendresse S, Craft S. Testosterone supplementation improves spatial and verbal memory in healthy older men. Neurology. 2001;57:80-88.

[99] Alexander GM, Swerdloff RS, Wang C, Davidson T, McDonald V, Steiner B, Hines M. Androgen-behavior correlations in hypogonadal men and eugonadal men (II. Cognitive Abilities). *Horm Behav*. 1998;33:85-94.

[100] Van Goozen SH, Cohen-Kettenis PT, Gooren LJ, Frijda NH, Van de Pol NE. Gender differences in behaviour: activating effects of cross-sex hormones. *Psychoneuroendocrinology*. 1995;20:343-363.

[101] Wolf OT, Preut R, Hellhammer DH, Kudielka BM, Schürmeyer TH, Kirschbaum C. Testosterone and cognition in elderly men: a single testosterone injection blocks the practice effect in verbal fluency, but has no effect on spatial or verbal memory. *Biol Psychiatry*. 2000;47:650-654.

[102] Salminen E, Portin R, Korpela J, Backman H, Parvinen LM, Helenius H, Nurmi M. Androgen deprivation and cognition in prostate cancer. *Br J Cancer*. 2003;89:971-976.

[103] Almeida OP, Waterreus, A, Spry N, Corica, T, Martins G, Martins RN, Flicker, L. Effect of testosterone deprivation on the cognitive performance of a patient with Alzheimer's Disease. *Int J Geriatr Psychiatry*. 2001; Aug 16(8): 823-5.
[104] Tenover JL. Testosterone and the aging male. *J Androl*. 1997;18:103-106.
[105] Okun MS, DeLongMR, Hanfelt J, Gearing M, Levey A. Plasma testosterone levels in Alzheimer and Parkinson diseases. *Neurology*. 2004;62:411-413.

In: Focus on Parkinson's Disease Research
Editor: Marianne J. Willow, pp. 65-78
ISBN 1-59454-924-9
© 2006 Nova Science Publishers, Inc.

Chapter IV

In Vivo Evaluation of Nigro-Striatal Dopaminergic Neuronal Function in Parkinson's Disease with Nuclear Medical Imaging Technology

Hideo Saji*[1,*]*, Hidekazu Kawashima*[1]*, Yasuhiko Iida*[1]*,
***Toshifumi Fukuoka*[2] *and Takayuki Iwaisako*[2]**
[1]Department of Patho-Functional Bioanalysis, Graduate School of Pharmaceutical Sciences, Kyoto University, Kyoto, Japan
[1]Environmental Health Science Laboratory, Sumitomo Chemical Co., Ltd., Konohana-ku, Osaka, Japan

Abstract

To elucidate the change in neuronal function with movement dysfunction occurring after the administration of a dopamine antagonist, the potency of high-resolution single photon emission computed tomography (SPECT) was estimated using an animal model in which Parkinsonian symptoms gradually progressed following chronic treatment with the antipsychotic haloperidol (HP).
A semi-quantitative SPECT analysis of brain dopaminergic synapses was combined with a motor behavior rating. Briefly, common marmosets were treated perorally with 1.25 mg/kg of HP twice a week for 6 months and adverse effects were monitored. Along with this scoring, SPECT was performed to evaluate the change in the striatal dopaminergic neurotransmission system. [^{123}I]2β-carbomethoxy-3β-(4-iodophenyl)tropane ([^{123}I]β-CIT) and [^{123}I](S)-(–)-3-iodo-2-hydroxy-6-methoxy-*N*-[(1-ethyl-2-pyrrolidinyl)methyl] benzamide ([^{123}I]IBZM) were used as radiolabeled ligands for the dopamine transporter

* Correspondence concerning this article should be addressed to Department of Patho-Functional Bioanalysis, Graduate School of Pharmaceutical Sciences, Kyoto University, 46-29 Yoshida-Shimoadachicho, Sakyo-ku, Kyoto 606-8501, Japan

(DAT) and dopamine D_2 receptor (D_2R), respectively. A SPECT image was obtained at 240 min and 60 min after the injection of 150 MBq of ligand, and then the amount of radioactivity (% injected dose/mL) in the striatum (Ac_{St}) and cerebellum (Ac_{Ce}) was measured. The ratio of Ac_{St} vs. Ac_{Ce} was calculated as an index of the binding potential of the ligands.

In the HP treatment group, dyskinetic behavior, such as abnormal gait and/or extension of limbs was elicited approximately 3 months after initial treatment, and the frequency continued to increase with time. On the other hand, changes in the SPECT image were observed prior to the manifestation of behavioral change: at 2 months, the specific accumulation of $[^{123}I]\beta$-CIT in the striatum had decreased to 0.8 of the level at commencement, and that of $[^{123}I]$IBZM had increased to 1.3. Both values continued to change with time, reaching 0.7 and 1.7 at 6 months, respectively. No behavioral or SPECT changes were observed in the placebo group.

Since HP is reported to be metabolized into 4-(4-chlorophenyl)-1-[4-(4-fluorophenyl)-4-oxobutyl]pyridinium ion (HPP^+), which has potential dopaminergic neurotoxicity, it was conceivable that chronic treatment with HP damaged neurons projecting from the substance nigra to striatum. So, the presynaptic changes observed with $[^{123}I]\beta$-CIT were considered to originate from this irreversible neurodegeneration. On the other hand, the increase in $[^{123}I]$IBZM suggested an upregulation of postsynaptic D_2R, following the presynaptic changes. These results suggested that, using noninvasive imaging techniques, dopaminergic neuronal change could be detected in Parkinsonian syndrome induced by long-term treatment with D_2R-binding antipsychotics.

Keywords: Tardive motor dysfunction, Dopamine transporter, Dopamine D2 receptor, Single photon emission computed tomography

INTRODUCTION

Parkinson's disease (PD) involves a progressive loss of motor dysfunction, and is clinically characterized by tremor, bradykinesia and persistent rigidity. In this disorder, a loss of dopaminergic neurons projecting from the substance nigra to striatum (A_9) results in a deficiency of dopamine (Bogerts *et al.*, 1983; Schultz, 1984; Scherman *et al.*, 1989).

For the *in vivo* assessment of dopaminergic neuronal functions in the brain, nuclear medical imaging techniques such as single photon emission computed tomography (SPECT) and positron emission tomography (PET) have often been applied. Using several radiolabeled tracers, functional changes in neurons were observed both in neurotoxin-treated animals (Brownell *et al.*, 2003; Saji *et al.*, 2003) and in PD patients (Booij *et al.*, 1999; Antonini *et al.*, 2003; Forsback *et al.*, 2004). It was reported that the accumulation of tracers was closely correlated with the stage of PD. Early noninvasive detection of PD, however, is required for beneficial therapy and improvements in quality of life. So, we prepared an animal model in which dopaminergic neuronal deficiency progresses gradually, and evaluated the process of functional change in the neurotransmission system using nuclear medical techniques.

Since typical antipsychotics block the dopamine D_2 receptor (D_2R), their use might contribute to the crisis of acute parkinsonism by affecting A_9 neurons (Reynolds, 1994; Kuenstler *et al.*, 1999; Blanchet, 2003). Haloperidol (HP), which is widely used to treat schizophrenic patients because of its antipsychotic potency, often induces parkinsonism, including tardive motor dysfunction (TMD). (Baldessarini *et al.*, 1979; Jenner *et al.*, 1985; Gerlach *et al.*, 1988; Beasley *et al.*, 1999). In the present study, the common marmoset was selected as a model for drug-induced PD because of its similarity to humans in terms of the selectivity of parkinsonism-inducing antipsychotics (Fukuoka *et al.*, 1997), and was treated long-term with oral HP.

The changes in dopaminergic neuronal transmission were evaluated *in vivo* using two SPECT radioligands; $[^{123}I]$-2β-carbomethoxy-3β-(4-iodophenyl)tropane ($[^{123}I]$β-CIT) for the dopamine transporter (DAT) and $[^{123}I]$-(S)-(–)-3-iodo-2-hydroxy-6-methoxy-N-[(1-ethyl-2-pyrrolidinyl)methyl]benzamide ($[^{123}I]$IBZM) for D_2R. Each SPECT analysis was performed in parallel with animal behavioral observations to elucidate the change in dopaminergic neuronal function during long-term treatment with D_2R-binding antipsychotics.

Materials and Methods

Animal experiments were conducted in accordance with our institutional guidelines, and the experimental procedures were approved by the Kyoto University Animal Care Committee.

Animal Preparation

Common marmosets (*Callithric jacchus*) weighing 370–445 g (bred by Japan E D M, Gifu, Japan) were housed individually in stainless steel cages in a temperature/humidity-controlled (28±2°C and 50±20%, respectively) animal room, on a balanced marmoset diet (CMS-1, CLEA Japan, Inc) with water *ad libitum*. HP (Research Biochemicals International: RBI, Natick, MA) was suspended in a 0.5% methylcellulose solution, and administered to the marmosets at 1.25 mg/kg twice weekly. Age-matched common marmosets (weighing 340–450 g) were administered vehicle (0.5% methylcellulose solution) as a control group. Animals were kept on the treatment schedule for 6 months.

Rating of Motor Activity

Common marmosets were observed in their home cages just before, and several times during the first 24 hr after, drug administration. All animals were examined for 5–7 min at each observation.

The observers recorded the frequency of HP-induced adverse effects referring to the criteria reported previously (Liebman *et al.*, 1980; Fukuoka *et al.*, 1997). Motor dysfunction was classified as abnormal gait (characterized by repeated circling, adducted hindlimbs, and elevated rump), abnormal behavior (persistent pushing of the head against the cage wall or ceiling), body writhing movement, persistent extension of limbs, and oral dyskinesia (abnormal tongue protrusions, licking movements, biting movements). Other neurological symptoms of motor behavior including tremors, catalepsy, sedation, blepharoptosis, hyperactivity, and reactions to observers were also recorded during each session. The scores except for catalepsy were as follows: 0 = signs absent (normal behavior); 1 = signs present once during each observation (4–6 min); 2 = signs repeatedly during each observation; and 3 = signs continuously present during each observation.

HPLC Systems for Radiolabeling

A SHIMADZU LC-6A, SPD-6A UV spectrophotometric detector (Shimadzu Co., Kyoto, Japan) attached to an Aloka NDW-351D NaI (Tl) scintillation radioisotope detector (Aloka Co., Ltd., Tokyo, Japan) was used in the following systems:

- System A: LICHROSORB RP18-5 (7.5×300 mm) column (Chemco Scientific Co., Ltd., Osaka, Japan), 75:25 (v/v) mixture of methanol and water containing 0.2% triethylamine, and a flow rate of 1.5 mL/min.
- System B: COSMOSIL 5C18-300 (10×250 mm) column (Nacalai Tesque Inc., Kyoto, Japan), 70:30 (v/v) mixture of methanol and water containing 0.2% triethylamine, and a flow rate of 3.0 mL/min.
- System C: COSMOSIL 5C18-AR-300 (4.6×150 mm) column (Nacalai Tesque), 70:30 (v/v) mixture of methanol and water containing 0.2% triethylamine, and a flow rate of 1.0 mL/min.

Radiolabeling Procedure for [^{123}I]β-CIT and [^{123}I]IBZM

The radioiodination of [^{123}I]2β-carbomethoxy-3β-(4-iodophenyl)tropane ([^{123}I]β-CIT), a ligand for DAT imaging, was accomplished with the oxidative alkylstannyl-[^{123}I]iodide exchange reaction as described previously (Zea-Ponce *et al.*, 1995) with slight modifications. Briefly, (2β-carbomethoxy-3β-(4-trimethylstannylphenyl)tropane (RBI) was reacted with no-carrier-added ammonium [^{123}I]iodide (Nihon Medi-Physics Co. Ltd., Hyogo, Japan). Hydrogen peroxide was used as an oxidizing agent. The reaction mixture was loaded onto a SEP-PAK C18 Cartridge (Waters Co., Milford, MA), and eluted with water, followed by ethanol to obtain [^{123}I]β-CIT. After evaporation, [^{123}I]β-CIT was dissolved finally into a solution of saline with 5% ethanol. The radiochemical purity of [^{123}I]β-CIT determined by reversed phase HPLC (System A) was greater than 95%. All radioactive compounds were eluted within 40 min after injection into the HPLC column. The total radiochemical yield was 55%.

[^{123}I]-(S)-(–)-3-Iodo-2-hydroxy-6-methoxy-N-[(1-ethyl-2-pyrrolidinyl)methyl]benzamide ([^{123}I]IBZM), a ligand for D_2R imaging, was radiosynthesized according to the chloramine T method reported previously (Kung *et al.*, 1989), with several modifications. Briefly, ((S)-(–)-2-hydroxy-6-methoxy-N-[(1-ethyl-2-pyrrolidinyl)methyl]benzamide (RBI) was reacted with no-carrier-added ammonium [^{123}I]iodide in the presence of chloramine T as the oxidant. The reaction mixture was then extracted with ethyl acetate. After evaporation, the residue was dissolved in methanol, and subjected to reversed phase HPLC purification (System B).

[^{123}I]IBZM was prepared for injection similarly to [^{123}I]β-CIT, and then analytical HPLC was performed (System C). The radiochemical purity was greater than 95%, and the total radiochemical yield was 30%.

Specific activity could not be directly measured with either ligand, but the theoretical value was 8.8 TBq/μmol.

SPECT Analysis

SPECT was performed before and 1, 2 and 6 months after initial HP treatment. During the period of the analysis, drug treatment was suspended. For imaging procedures, the anesthetic consisted of a ketamine-xylazine cocktail (20 mg/kg and 3 mg/kg, respectively, i.m.), followed by pentobarbital sodium (20 mg/kg, i.p.). All animals received a single bolus of [^{123}I]β-CIT (150–200 MBq) into the saphenous vein, and 4 hr later, data acquisition was started as dynamic SPECT scans (360° rotation, 40 sec/frame for 32 frames), using a SPECT2000H-40 gamma camera (Hitachi Medical Co., Tokyo, Japan) with specially designed pinhole collimators (30% window; 159 keV energy peak; 128×128 matrix mode; pixel size of 1.33 mm) connected on-line to an RW-3000 data processor as reported previously (Ishizu *et al.*, 1995). After one week, no radioactivity in animals was detected, then [^{123}I]IBZM (150–200 MBq) was injected in the same manner as [^{123}I]β-CIT. SPECT scanning was similarly performed from 1 hr after the injection.

In the dynamic study, five consecutive slices (for a total slice thickness of 3.85 mm) of the brain were used for data analysis. Regions of interest (ROIs) were drawn onto the left and right striatum (St) and onto the cerebellum (Ce) in the sagittal and/or transaxial MR images obtained with UNITY plus 300WB (Varian, Inc, Palo Alto, CA). The accumulation of radioactivity at each ROI, ac_{St} and ac_{Ce} (% injected dose/mL), was measured, after which the value of

$$(ac_{St} - ac_{Ce})/ac_{Ce} = ac_{St}/ac_{Ce} - 1$$

was calculated as the Binding Ratio (BR) (Asenbaum *et al.*, 1997). Since ac_{St} and ac_{Ce} were regarded as the total binding and nondisplaceable uptake (free + nonspecific binding) of the radioligand, respectively, ac_{St} minus ac_{Ce} corresponded to the specific binding of radioligands in the striatal area. Consequently, BR indicated specific binding/nondisplaceable uptake, which was proportional to binding potential (B_{max}/K_d) (Laruelle *et al.*, 1994, 2000; Malison *et al.*, 1998; Anand *et al.*, 2000).

Statistical Analysis

In the SPECT analysis, calculated values were compared between vehicle-treated and HP-treated groups using independent *t*-tests.

Measurement of HPP^+ in the Tissue of a HP-Treated Animal

A common marmoset was administered perorally with 1.25 mg/kg of HP, and sacrificed 3 hr later. The brain was dissected, and HP metabolites were extracted as reported previously (Igarashi et al., 1992). Briefly, tissue was homogenized in a 1.15% KCl solution with a Polytron homogenizer, mixed with an equal volume of methanol containing 2% acetic acid to sediment protein, and centrifuged at 10,000 *g* for 10 min. The supernatant was obtained as a sample.

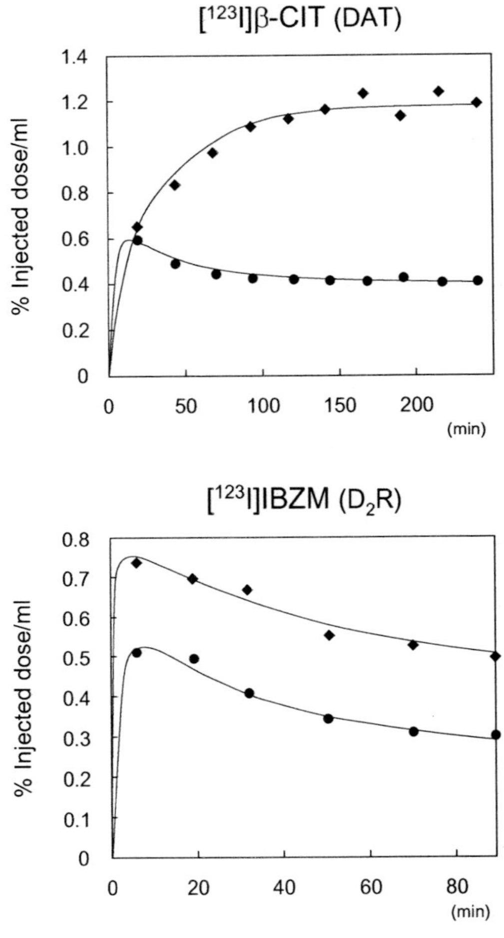

Figure 1. Time-activity curves of regional accumulation in common marmoset brain. SPECT imaging was performed repeatedly from 15 min to 240 min ([^{123}I]β-CIT) or 90 min ([^{123}I]IBZM) after injection with a dose of 150 MBq each. (A) [^{123}I]β-CIT accumulated in the striatal region (◆), but was washed out fast from the cerebellar region (●). (B) [^{123}I]IBZM accumulated immediately after injection, with gradual decreases in both regions of interest (ROIs), striatal (◆) and cerebellar (●), defined in Figure 2.

A quantitative analysis of HPP^+ was performed with reference to the HPLC method reported by Igarashi et al., with some modifications. A SHIMADZU PF-10A$_{XL}$ fluorescence detector (302 nm excitation / 370 nm emission) (Shimadzu Co., Kyoto, Japan) was connected to a YMC-Pack Pro C18 (4.6×150 mm) column (YMC Co., Ltd., Kyoto, Japan), and a 40:60

(v/v) mixture of acetonitrile and 10 mM phosphate buffer (pH 3.0, containing 5 mM sodium 1-octanesulfonate) was delivered at a flow rate of 1.0 mL/min.

RESULTS

SPECT Measurement of $[^{123}I]\beta$-CIT and $[^{123}I]$IBZM Binding

To evaluate $[^{123}I]\beta$-CIT and $[^{123}I]$IBZM kinetics in the brain, each ligand was injected into normal common marmosets, and then the regional accumulation of radioactivity was measured by SPECT to prepare a time-activity curve (Fig. 1). Imaging was performed from 15 min to 240 min after injection for $[^{123}I]\beta$-CIT and to 90 min for $[^{123}I]$IBZM. Since it was reported that dopaminergic synapses are present at high density in the striatum but at low density in the cerebellum, regions of interest (ROIs) were drawn onto the striatum and cerebellum, and the radioactivity in these two areas, ac_{St} and ac_{Ce} (% injected dose/mL), was measured. Since the accumulation at the bilateral striatum was approximately equivalent for each radioligand, ac_{St} was calculated as an average for the two sites. In the striatum, the amount of $[^{123}I]\beta$-CIT activity increased gradually and reached a plateau at about 180 min postinjection. In the cerebellum, a similar accumulation of radioactivity was observed immediately after injection, but it was washed out and reached a constant value 150 min after injection. $[^{123}I]$IBZM showed a rapid accumulation and slow clearance in both regions. However, the clearance rate was lower in the striatum than cerebellum. The ratio of *in vivo* specific binding of the radioligand (ac_{St} minus ac_{Ce}) to nondisplaceable uptake (ac_{Ce}), i.e. BR, became constant at 240 min and 60 min after injection of $[^{123}I]\beta$-CIT and $[^{123}I]$IBZM, respectively. Therefore, these points were set up as acquisition times to gain the data for BR. The values of the two radioligands immediately before the drug treatment study were 1.06±0.23 vs. 0.28±0.06 for $[^{123}I]\beta$-CIT (ac_{St} and ac_{Ce}, respectively) and 0.59±0.14 vs. 0.34±0.07 for $[^{123}I]$IBZM. The calculated BR value was 2.84±0.41 ($[^{123}I]\beta$-CIT) and 0.76±0.18 ($[^{123}I]$IBZM).

Time-Dependent Changes in Dopaminergic Neuronal Activity

Figure 2 shows (A) a typical sagittal brain image at 240 min after the injection of $[^{123}I]\beta$-CIT into an animal and (B) an MR image corresponding to the SPECT image, which was used for determination of striatum (St) and cerebellum (Ce) regions in the merged image (Fig. 2C). High levels of radioligand had clearly accumulated in the striatum. A similar image was obtained after the injection of $[^{123}I]$IBZM. No significant differences in levels of radioactivity were observed between the right and left striatum.

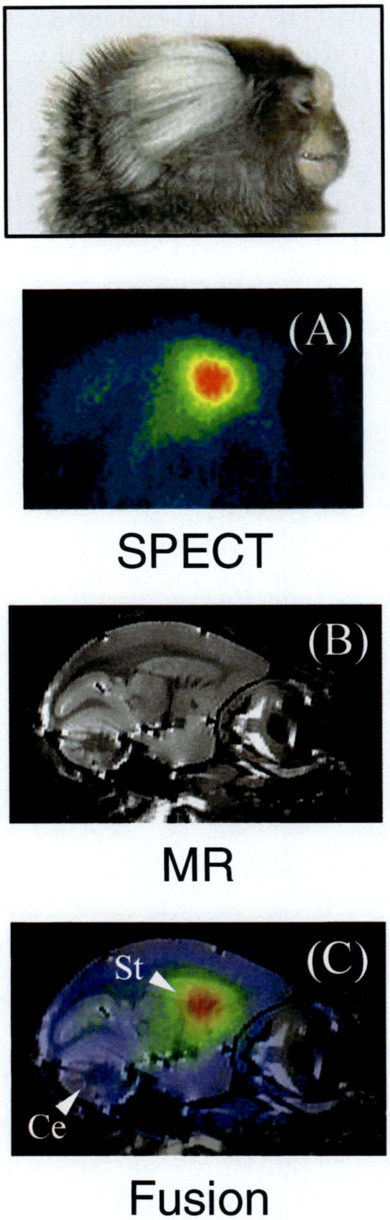

Figure 2. Representative images of common marmoset brain. (A) A sagittal SPECT image from dynamic scan post-administration of 150 MBq of [^{123}I]β-CIT (229 to 251 min). (B) An MR image for defining regions of interest (ROIs) in the striatum (St) and cerebellum (Ce). (C) A SPECT image (A) superimposed on an MR image (B). Striatal uptake is clearly depicted as indicated by the arrowhead (▷). Similar images were obtained after injection of [^{123}I]IBZM.

In Figure 3, BR values of [^{123}I]β-CIT and [^{123}I]IBZM were measured at 1, 2 and 6 months after the commencement of treatment with (A) vehicle and (B) HP, and then values relative to each pretreatment value were plotted as the "Relative Binding Ratio" (RBR) together with the score related to symptoms of dyskinesia. In the HP treatment group, dyskinetic symptoms (especially abnormal gait and extension of limbs) were obvious 2 to 3 months after the initial administration. The score increased with time, and 5 months later, the animals showed constant motor dysfunction. A significant decrease in the RBR of [^{123}I]β-CIT was confirmed at 2 months (1.00±0.07 vs. 0.82±0.07 in groups treated with vehicle and HP, respectively; means ± SD, n=4–6) (P<0.01) and 6 months (0.99±0.07 vs. 0.70±0.05, n=5–6) (P<0.0001) after the initial administration. In contrast, the RBR of [^{123}I]IBZM was increased at each time point (0.97±0.07 vs. 1.33±0.10 in groups treated with vehicle and HP for 2 months, respectively; means ± SD, n=4–6) (P=0.0001), (1.04±0.07 vs. 1.66±0.11, 6 months, n=5–6) (P<0.0001). No change was observed in the vehicle-treated controls.

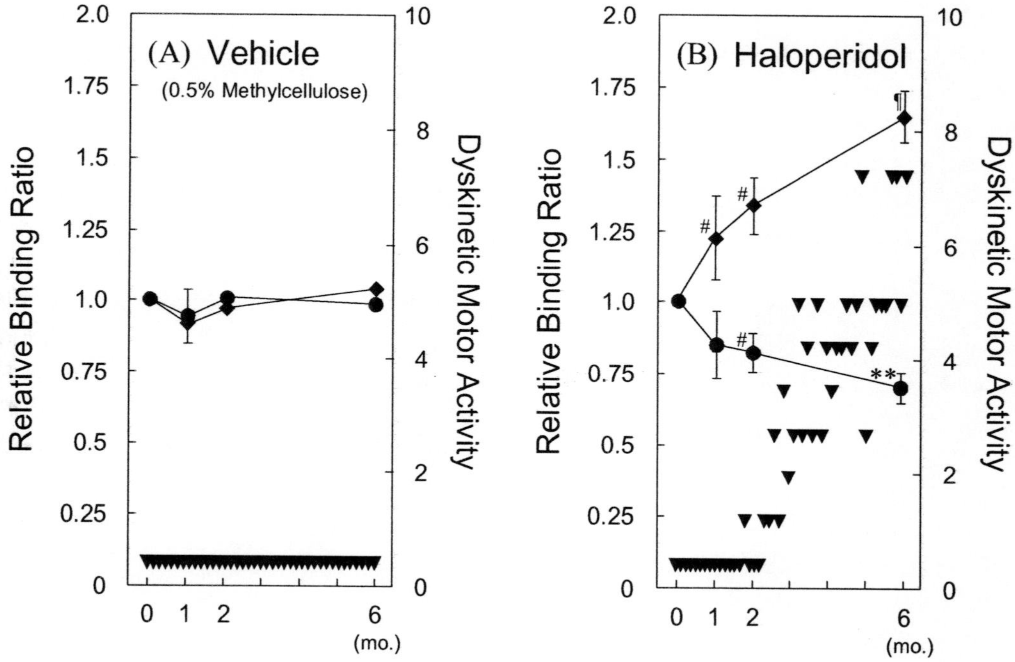

Figure 3. Relationship between functional changes in brain dopaminergic neuronal transmission expressed as a Relative Binding Ratio (RBR) and locomotor activity expressed as Dyskinetic Motor Activity, as described under methods. Common marmosets were treated perorally with (A) 1 mL/kg of 0.5% methylcellulose as vehicle alone (n=6) and (B) 1.25 mg/kg of haloperidol (n=5) twice a week. Neuronal activity measured by SPECT using [^{123}I]β-CIT (●) and [^{123}I]IBZM (◆) before (0 month) and 1, 2 and 6 months after commencement of treatment. Left ordinate: RBR (values relative to 0 month). Right ordinate: Dyskinetic Motor Activity score (▼). # *P*<0.05; ** *P*<0.005, ¶ *P*<0.001, compared with 0 month.

Quantitative Analysis of HPP$^+$

Using HPLC, HPP$^+$ was detected in the brain (21.5 nmol/g wet tissue) and plasma (62.4 nmol/mL) samples of a common marmoset at 3 hr after the peroral administration of 1.25 mg/kg of HP.

DISCUSSION

Changes in dopaminergic neuronal transmission in the brain have been reported in animal models of PD. In many cases, the lesions were produced rapidly by a potent neurotoxin, such as 6-hydroxydopamine or 1-methyl-4-phenyl-1,2,3,6-tetrahydropyridine (MPTP) (Nagatsu, 1990; Wesemann *et al.*, 1993; Amalric *et al.*, 1995; Ben *et al.*, 1999; Doudet *et al.*, 2002). In general, however, PD progresses gradually. Thus, to investigate the neuronal changes leading to PD, we attempted to use a model in which Parkinsonian symptoms develop gradually. Namely, in this study, we employed chronic treatment with HP, which induces a gradual PD-like tardive motor dysfunction (TMD).

Since the manifestations of drug-induced parkinsonism frequently show species-specific and individual differences, the selection of experimental animal species and the simultaneous measurement of behavior with dopaminergic neuronal activity in the same animal are important. Thus, the common marmoset was selected as an experimental model because of its similarity to humans with regard to the selectivity of parkinsonism-inducing antipsychotics, and the brain dopaminergic neurotransmission function was noninvasively evaluated by SPECT in combination with pharmacological observations.

To perform a semiquantitative analysis of dopaminergic neurotransmission using SPECT, ROIs were set on the striatum, a region with a high density of DAT and dopamine receptors, and the cerebellum, a region with a very low density of DAT and dopamine receptors (Fig. 2) (Palacios *et al.*, 1988; De Keyser *et al.*, 1989; Brücke *et al.*, 1993). Although [^{123}I]β-CIT also has moderate affinity for the serotonin transporter (SERT), SERT is distributed in the striatum at a much lower density than DAT, and therefore, the striatal-specific accumulation of [^{123}I]β-CIT is considered to be due to the density of DAT (Laruelle *et al.*, 1993). Furthermore, since the nondisplaceable uptake in the striatum was assumed to be comparable with that in the cerebellum (ac_{Ce}), the specific binding in the striatum was calculated by subtracting the concentration of radioactivity in the cerebellum from that in the striatum. Therefore, the specific to nondisplaceable ratio in the striatum (BR) was regarded as an index of the binding potential (B_{max}/K_d), that is, the ligand affinity and/or density of DAT or D_2R in this region. In many studies using neurolytic animal models, it has been demonstrated that the changes in tracer accumulation are linked to receptor density (B_{max}) (Liberini *et al.*, 1995; Ambardekar *et al.*, 1999; Barc *et al.*, 2002), consequently, the BR values observed in this SPECT study were considered to be due to the density of DAT or D_2R, although additional investigations are needed.

RBR with [^{123}I]β-CIT and [^{123}I]IBZM revealed that the animals with long-term HP treatment showed a significant decrease of DAT and significant increase of D_2R density in the striatum with time (Fig. 3). Through a combination of SPECT and the rating of pharmacological behavior, it was proved that the abnormality of brain dopaminergic neurotransmission induced by HP treatment is involved in the manifestation of TMD. Given that dyskinetic behavior was observed later than the change in the accumulation of radioligand (Fig. 3), neuronal changes preceding motor dysfunction could be detected *in vivo* using an appropriate tracer.

The cause of the TMD induced by the treatment with HP is unclear. However, studies on MPTP, a typical dopaminergic neurotoxin, showed that it undergoes oxidization into 1-

methyl-4-phenylpyridinium ion (MPP^+), followed by uptake into dopaminergic neurons via DAT, resulting in selective neurotoxicity (Saporito *et al.*, 1991; Tipson *et al.*, 1993). Thus, the toxicity of several compounds possessing structural similarity to MPP^+ has been investigated, and recently, 4-(4-Chlorophenyl)-1-[4-(4-fluorophenyl)-4-oxobutyl]pyridinium ion (HPP^+), a pyridinium metabolite of HP, was reported as a candidate (Subramanyam *et al.*, 1991; Usuki *et al.*, 1998). Namely, studies *in vitro* have shown that HPP^+ possesses dopaminergic neurotoxicity (Bloomquist *et al.*, 1994; Fang *et al.*, 1995). Moreover, HP treatment induced morphological impairment in nigro-striatal DA neurons (Marchese *et al.*, 2002). Though less toxic than MPP^+, HPP^+ might contribute to some extrapyramidal side effect induced by the treatment with HP.

In this study, HPP^+ was detected in the brain of common marmoset administered HP. This finding suggests that irreversible damage to nigro-striatal dopaminergic neurons caused by HPP^+ result in a decrease in the density of DAT and the $[^{123}I]\beta$-CIT level in the striatum might decrease.

On the other hand, the uptake of $[^{123}I]$IBZM in the striatum was increased. This is probably due to an upregulation of D_2R to compensate for the reduced dopamine concentration in the synaptic cleft of lesioned presynaptic neurons and/or D_2R blockade by HP.

In conclusion, the present study demonstrated that an increase of D_2R and decrease of DAT occurred in the striatal region in common marmosets treated chronically with HP. Furthermore, the results suggested that the imaging *in vivo* of cerebral dopaminergic neuronal function with nuclear medical imaging technology might have potential applications for the early detection of PD.

ACKNOWLEDGEMENTS

We would like to thank Nihon Medi-Physics Co., Ltd., Hyogo, Japan, for providing ammonium $[^{123}I]$iodide.

REFERENCES

Amalric M, Moukhles H, Nieoullon A, Daszuta A. (1995) Complex deficits on reaction time performance following bilateral intrastriatal 6-OHDA infusion in the rat. *Eur J Neurosci 7*: 972–980

Ambardekar AV, Ilinsky IA, Forestl W, Bowery NG, Kultas-Ilinsky K. (1999) Distribution and properties of $GABA_B$ antagonist $[^3H]$CGP 62349 binding in the rhesus monkey thalamus and basal ganglia and the influence of lesions in the reticular thalamic nucleus. *Neuroscience 93*: 1339–1347

Anand A, Verhoeff P, Seneca N, Zoghbi SS, Seibyl JP, Charney DS, Innis RB. (2000) Brain SPECT imaging of amphetamine-induced dopamine release in euthymic bipolar disorder patients. *Am J Psychiatry 157*: 1108-1114

Antonini A, Benti R, De Notaris R, Tesei S, Zecchinelli A, Sacilotto G, Meucci N, Canesi M, Mariani C, Pezzoli G, Gerundini P. (2003) ^{123}I-Ioflupane/SPECT binding to striatal dopamine transporter (DAT) uptake in patients with Parkinson's disease, multiple system atrophy, and progressive supranuclear plasy. *Neurol Sci 24*: 149–150

Asenbaum S, Brücke T, Pirker W, Podreka I, Angelberger P, Wenger S, Wöber C, Müller C, Deecke L. (1997) Imaging of dopamine transporters with iodine-123-beta-CIT and SPECT in Parkinson's disease. *J Nucl Med 38*: 1–6

Baldessarini RJ, Tarsy D. (1979) Relationship of the actions of neuroleptic drugs to the pathophysiology of tardive dyskinesia. *Int Rev Neurobiol 21*: 1–44

Barc S, Page G, Barrier L, Garreau L, Guilloteau D, Fauconneau B, Chalon S. (2002) Relevance of different striatal markers in assessment of the MPP^+-induced dopaminergic nigrostriatal injury in rat. *J Neurochem 80*: 365–374

Beasley CM, Dellva MA, Tamura RN, Morgenstern H, Glazer WM, Ferguson K, Tollefson GD. (1999) Randomised double-blind comparison of the incidence of tardive dyskinesia in patients with schizophrenia during long-term treatment with olanzapine or haloperidol. *Br J Psychiatry 174*: 23–30

Ben V, Blin O, Bruguerolle B. (1999) Time-dependent striatal dopamine depletion after injection of 6-hydroxydopamine in the rat. Comparison of single bilateral and double bilateral lesions. *J Pharm Pharmacol 51*: 1405–1408

Blanchet PJ. (2003) Antipsychotic drug-induced movement disorders. *Can J Neurol Sci 30 Suppl 1*: S101–107

Bloomquist J, King E, Wright A, Mytilineou C, Kimura K, Castagnoli K, Castagnoli N Jr. (1994) 1-Methyl-4-phenylpyridinium-like neurotoxicity of a pyridinium metabolite derived from haloperidol: cell culture and neurotransmitter uptake studies. *J Pharmacol Exp Ther 270*: 822–830

Bogerts B, Hantsch J, Herzer M. (1983) A morphometric study of the dopamine-containing cell groups in the mesencephalon of normals, Parkinson patients, and schizophrenics. *Biol Psychiatry 18*: 951–969

Booij J, Tissingh G, Winogrodzka A, van Royen EA. (1999) Imaging of the dopaminergic neurotransmission system using single-photon emission tomography and positron emission tomography in patients with parkinsonism. *Eur J Nucl Med 26*: 171–182

Brownell A-L, Canales K, Chen YI, Jenkins BG, Owen C, Livni E, Yu M, Cicchetti F, Sanchez-Pernaute R, Isacson O. (2003) Mapping of brain function after MPTP-induced neurotoxicity in a primate Parkinson's disease model. *Neuroimage 20*: 1064–1075

Brücke T, Kornhuber J, Angelberger P, Asenbaum S, Frassine H, Podreka I. (1993) SPECT imaging of dopamine and serotonin transporters with [^{123}I]β-CIT. Binding kinetics in the human brain. *J Neural Transm Gen Sect 94*: 137–146

De Keyser J, De Backer JP, Ebinger G, Vauquelin G. (1989) [^{3}H]GBR 12935 binding to dopamine uptake sites in the human brain. *J Neurochem 53:* 1400–1404

Doudet DJ, Holden JE, Jivan S, McGeer E, Wyatt RJ. (2000) In vivo PET studies of the dopamine D2 receptors in rhesus monkeys with long-term MPTP-induced parkinsonism. *Synapse 38*: 105–113

Fang J, Zuo D, Yu PH. (1995) Comparison of cytotoxicity of a quaternary pyridinium metabolite of haloperidol (HP^+) with neurotoxin N-methyl-4-phenylpyridinium (MPP^+) towards cultured dopaminergic neuroblastoma cells. *Psychopharmacology 121*: 373–378

Forsback S, Niemi R, Marjamäki P, Eskola O, Bergman J, Grönroos T, Haaparanta M, Haapalinna A, Rinne J, Solin O. (2004) Uptake of 6-[^{18}F]fluoro-L-dopa and [^{18}F]CFT reflect nigral neuronal loss in a rat model of Parkinson's disease. *Synapse 51*: 119–127

Fukuoka T, Nakano M, Kohda A, Okuno Y, Matsuo M. (1997) The common marmoset (*Callithrix jacchus*) as a model for neuroleptic-induced acute dystonia. *Pharmacol Biochem Behav 58*: 947–953

Gerlach J, Casey DE. (1988) Tardive dyskinesia. *Acta Psych Scand 77*: 369–378

Igarashi K, Castagnoli N. Jr. (1992) Determination of the pyridinium metabolite derived from haloperidol in brain tissue, plasma and urine by high-performance liquid chromatography with fluorescence detection. *J Chromatograph 579*: 277–283

Ishizu K, Mukai T, Yonekura Y, Pagani M, Fujita T, Magata Y, Nishizawa S, Tamaki N, Shibasaki H, Konishi J. (1995) Ultra-high resolution SPECT system using four pinhole collimators for small animal studies. *J Nucl Med 36:* 2282–2287

Jenner P, Rupniak NM, Marsden CD. (1985) Differential alteration of striatal D-1 and D-2 receptors induced by the long-term administration of haloperidol, sulpiride or clozapine to rats. *Psychopharmacology Suppl 2*: 174–181

Kuenstler U, Juhnhold U, Knapp WH, Gertz HJ. (1999) Positive correlation between reduction of handwriting area and D_2 dopamine receptor occupancy during treatment with neuroleptic drugs. *Psychiatry Res 90*: 31–39

Kung MP, Kung HF. (1989) Peracetic acid as a superior oxidant for preparation of [^{123}I]IBZM: a potential dopamine D-2 receptor imaging agent. *J Labeled Compd Radipharm 27*: 691–700

Laruelle M, Baldwin RM, Malison RT, Zea-Ponce Y, Zoghbi SS, Al-Tikriti MS, Sybirska EH, Zimmermann RC, Wisniewski G, Neumeyer JL, Milius RA, Wang S, Smith EO, Roth RH, Charney DS, Hoffer PB, Innis RB. (1993) SPECT imaging of dopamine and serotonin transporters with [^{123}I]β-CIT: pharmacological characterization of brain uptake in nonhuman primates. *Synapse 13*: 295–309

Laruelle M, Wallace E, Seibyl J, Baldwin R, Zea-Ponce Y, Zoghbi S, Neumeyer J, Charney D, Hoffer P, Innis R. (1994) Graphical, kinetic, and equilibrium analyses of in vivo [^{123}I]β-CIT binding to dopamine transporters in healthy human subjects. *J Cereb Blood Flow Metab 14*: 982–994

Laruelle M, Abi-Dargham A, Van Dyck C, Gil R, D'Souza DC, Krystal J, Seibyl J, Baldwin R, Innis R. (2000) Dopamine and serotonin transporters in patients with schizophrenia: an imaging study with [^{123}I]β-CIT. *Biol Psychiatry 47*: 371–379

Liberini P, Reuben M, Clarke PB, Cuello AC. (1995) Nerve growth factor treatment restores [^{3}H]QNB binding site density in adult rat subjected to cortical infarction. *Neuroreport 15*: 419–420

Liebman JM, Neale R. (1980) Neuroleptic-induced acute dyskinesias in squirrel monkeys: Correlation with propensity to cause extrapyramidal side effects. *Psychopharmacology 68*: 25–29

Malison RT, McCance E, Carpenter LL, Baldwin RM, Seibyl JP, Price LH, Kosten TR, Innis RB. (1998) [^{123}I]β-CIT SPECT imaging of dopamine transporter availability after mazindol administration in human cocaine addicts. *Psychopharmacology 137*: 321–325

Marchese G, Casu MA, Bartholini F, Ruiu S, Saba P, Gessa GL, Pani L. (2002) Sub-chronic treatment with classical but not atypical antipsychotics produces morphological changes in rat nigro-striatal dopaminergic neurons directly related to "early onset" vacuous chewing. *Eur J Neurosci 15*: 1187–1196

Nagatsu T. (1990) Change of tyrosine hydroxylase in the parkinsonian brain and in the brain of MPTP-treated mice as revealed by homospecific activity. *Neurochem Res 15*: 425–429

Palacios JM, Camp M, Cortés R, Probst A. (1988) Mapping dopamine receptors in the human brain. *J Neural Transm Suppl 27*: 227–235

Reynolds GP. (1994) Antipsychotic drug mechanisms and neurotransmitter systems in schizophrenia. *Acta Psychiatr Scand Suppl 380*: 36–40

Saji H, Iida Y, Kawashima H, Ogawa M, Kitamura Y, Mukai T, Shimazu S, Yoneda F. (2003) *In vivo* imaging of brain dopaminergic neurotransmission system in small animals with high-resolution single photon emission computed tomography. *Anal Sci 19*: 67–71

Saporito MS, Heikkila RE, Youngser SK, Nicklas WJ, Herbert MG. (1991) Dopaminergic neurotoxicity of 1-methyl-4-phenylpiridinium analogs in cultured neurons: relationship to the dopamine uptake system and inhibition of mitochondrial respiration. *J Pharmacol Exp Ther 260:* 1400–1409

Scherman D, Desnos C, Darchen F, Pollak P, Javoy-Agid F, Agid Y. (1989) Striatal dopamine deficiency in Parkinson's disease: role of aging. *Ann Neurol 26*: 551–557

Schultz W. (1984) Recent physiological and pathophysiological aspects of Parkinsonian movement disorders. *Life Sci 34*: 2213–2223

Subramanyam B, Woolf T, Castagnoli N Jr. (1991) Studies on the in vitro conversion of haloperidol to a potentially neurotoxic pyridinium metabolite. *Chem Res Toxicol 4:* 123–128

Tipson KF, Singer TP. (1993) Advances in our understanding of the mechanisms of the neurotoxicity of MPTP and related compounds. *J Neurochem 61*: 1191–1206

Usuki E, Van der Schyf CJ, Castagnoli N Jr. (1998) Metabolism of haloperidol and its tetrahydropyridine dehydration product HPTP. *Drug Metab Rev 30*: 809–826

Wesemann W, Grote C, Clement HW, Block F, Sontag KH. (1993) Functional studies on monoaminergic transmitter release in parkinsonism. *Prog Neuropsychopharmacol Biol Psychiatry 17*: 487–499

Zea-Ponce Y, Baldwin RM, Laruelle M, Wang S, Naumeyer IL, Innis RB. (1995) Simplified multidose preparation of iodine-123-β-CIT: a marker for dopamine transporters. *J Nucl Med 36*: 525–529

In: Focus on Parkinson's Disease Research
Editor: Marianne J. Willow, pp. 79-96
ISBN 1-59454-924-9
© 2006 Nova Science Publishers, Inc.

Chapter V

PARKINSON'S DISEASE – USING DRUG THERAPY TO SLOW DOWN DISEASE PROGRESSION

James David Adams*, Jun Yang and Lori Klaidman
USC School of Pharmacy, Los Angeles, CA

ABSTRACT

Parkinson's disease is a progressive neurodegenerative disease involving loss of dopaminergic neurons in the substantia nigra of the midbrain. Dopaminergic neurons appear to die by a process of necrosis or apoptosis that is induced by oxidative stress. Oxygen radicals abstract hydrogen from DNA forming DNA radicals that lead to DNA fragmentation, activation of DNA protective mechanisms, NAD depletion and necrosis or apoptosis. Oxygen radicals can be formed in dopaminergic neurons by redox cycling of MPP^+, the active metabolite of MPTP. This redox cycling mechanism involves the reduction of MPP^+ by a number of enzymes, especially flavin containing enzymes, some of which are found in mitochondria. Tyrosine hydroxylase is present in all dopaminergic neurons and is involved in the synthesis of dopamine. However, tyrosine hydroxylase can form oxygen radicals in a redox mechanism involving its cofactor, tetrahydrobiopterin. Levodopa is a precursor for dopamine, an inhibitor of tyrosine hydroxylase, and prolongs patient's lives. Dopamine may be oxidized by monoamine oxidase to form oxygen radicals and 3,4-dihydroxyphenylacetaldehyde. Selegiline is a monoamine oxidase inhibitor used in Parkinson's disease. Selegiline may be able to slow down the progression of the disease. 3,4-Dihydroxyphenylacetaldehyde may be oxidized by aldehyde dehydrogenase with the formation of oxygen radicals and 3,4-dihydroxyphenylacetic acid. Aldehyde dehydrogenase inhibitors are not used in Parkinson's disease. There is, however, a theoretical basis for the use of aldehyde

* Correspondence concerning this article should be addressed to Dr. James David Adams USC School of Pharmacy, 1985 Zonal Avenue, PSC 508, Los Angeles, CA 90089-9121. Tel: (323) 442-1362. Email: jadams@usc.edu.

dehydrogenase inhibitors to slow down the progression of the disease. Future treatment of Parkinson's disease could consider the inhibition of oxygen radical formation in dopaminergic neurons or ways to stimulate DNA repair and prevent cell death.

Keywords: tyrosine hydroxylase, aldehyde dehydrogenase, nicotinamide, monoamine oxidase

ABBREVIATIONS

ALDH – aldehyde dehydrogenase
DHP – 1-methyl-4-phenyl-1,4-dihydropyridine
DOPAC – 3,4-dihydroxyphenylacetic acid
DOPAL – 3,4-dihydroxyphenylacetaldehyde
MAO – monoamine oxidase
$MPDP^+$ - 1-methyl-4-phenyl-2,3-dihydropyridine
MPP^+ - 1-methyl-4-phenylpyridine
MPTP – 1-methyl-4-phenyl-1,2,3,6-tetrahydropyridine
TH – tyrosine hydroxylase

INTRODUCTION

Parkinson's disease is a progressive disease that occurs most frequently after the age of 65. The disease slowly progresses until the patient is not able to move normally and eventually dies. It is not clear if the loss of dopaminergic neurons or some other cause leads to the death of these patients. Drug therapy is effective at helping patients in the early stages of the disease [1,2]. However, as the disease progresses, drug therapy becomes less effective. It is important to emphasize that drug therapy with levodopa helps prolong the lives of patients with Parkinson's disease. Therefore, the drugs used in Parkinson's disease may be neuroprotective agents that protect the brain from the damaging effects of the disease [1].

Parkinson's disease is caused by the death of dopaminergic neurons in the midbrain, a heavily pigmented region of the human brain. Therefore, the loss of dopaminergic neurons is accompanied by the loss of the pigment. These cells are killed by a process of oxidative stress wherein oxygen radicals are generated in the neurons. Of course, oxygen radicals are formed constantly in every cell of the body. The major source of oxygen radicals in dopaminergic neurons is not clear, but for years has been assumed to be the nonenzymatic oxidation of dopamine. The dopaminergic neurons of the midbrain may become unable to effectively protect themselves from oxygen radicals. This may allow the damaging effects of oxygen radicals to accumulate until the neurons die. It is very important to find out which of the defense mechanisms is compromised in dopaminergic neurons that are destined to die. It is known that aging makes DNA more susceptible to fragmentation induced by oxygen radicals [3]. A careful examination of the mechanisms involved in this increased susceptibility might lead to drug therapy to enhance protective mechanisms and slow down the progression of the disease.

Mitochondrial dysfunction and complex 1 inhibition have been implicated in Parkinson's disease. This dysfunction may lead to oxygen radical formation and the loss of the mitochondrion. It appears that oxygen radicals formed by mitochondria may have little effect on cell death induced by nuclear DNA damage under normal conditions [4]. Mitochondria are made and replaced in dopaminergic neurons on a constant basis. The loss of a portion of the mitochondria in a cell may not be critical.

There are several other mechanisms of oxygen radical formation in dopaminergic neurons. For instance iron in the midbrain may catalyze the formation of oxygen radicals [5]. In addition, dopamine may oxidize, nonenzymatically, forming oxygen radicals and various oxidation products of dopamine such as various quinones and neuromelanin [6]. Neuromelanin may be the major pigment of dopaminergic neurons. These mechanisms have been extensively explored and reviewed [7,8].

Does dopamine autoxidation explain the progression of Parkinson's disease? The answer is clearly no. Levodopa therapy prolongs the lives of patients [9,10,11]. Levodopa is a precursor for dopamine and increases dopamine turnover in the brain. If dopamine autoxidation were critical to disease progression, levodopa treated patients would die faster than untreated patients. However, levodopa has the potential to induce toxicity after many years of use in the midbrain that may limit the use of levodopa as discussed below.

The dopamine autoxidation theory has lead to the exploration of antioxidant compounds in the treatment of Parkinson's disease. The strategy has been to protect lipids in the cell membranes of dopaminergic neurons from lipid peroxidation. So far, none of the potential antioxidants has been approved for use in the US. This includes vitamin E, which is a very potent inhibitor of lipid peroxidation. None of the potential antioxidants have shown significant clinical effects in Parkinson's disease, except for exifone, a benzophenone antioxidant, that proved to be hepatotoxic [1]. This could be because protecting lipids is not the critical mechanism in Parkinson's disease.

New dopaminergic agonists, pramipexole and ropinirole, are now being used as the first therapy in Parkinson's disease or as adjuncts to levodopa [12,13,14]. There is preliminary evidence that these agents may be neuroprotective and may be able to slow down disease progression in patients [15,16,17]. However, longevity studies in patients must be done to see if they really extend the lives of patients. Dopamine agonists may be able to interact with presynaptic D_2 autoreceptors and decrease dopamine release. This may slow down dopamine turnover, which could theoretically decrease oxygen radical formation. Levodopa, but to a much lesser extent pramipexole, appears to be able to down regulate the synthesis of the dopamine transporter [18]. This down regulation artifactually makes disease progression appear to be faster in levodopa therapy, at least in PET studies. This dopamine transporter effect artifactually makes pramipexole appear to be neuroprotective in comparison to levodopa. Ropinirole effects on dopa decarboxylase, dopa uptake systems and other enzymes are not known. These enzymes are critical in Parkinson's disease. Despite reported neuroprotection during five year studies with ropinirole and pramipexole, the motor scores of patients were not better, or even worse, than levodopa treated patients [18]. Surely, five years of neuroprotection should have produced better motor scores in dopamine agonist treated patients compared to levodopa treated patients. However, patients maintained on pramipexole or ropinirole have a delayed requirement for levodopa therapy. This implies that pramipexole and ropinirole are capable of slowing down disease progression. Longevity studies are required to see if they really do slow down the disease.

Despite the possible neuroprotective mechanisms of pramipexole and ropinirole, they have toxicity problems in patients. Both ropinirole and pramipexole induce orthostatic hypotension and dizziness [19]. This may lead to falling, hip fracture and potential death of patients. Both of these powerful dopaminergic agonists are potent hallucinogens and induce hallucinations in a large portion of patients [20]. These hallucinations can make caring for these patients a problem. In addition, the effects of dopamine agonists appear to wane within a few years [21]. It appears to be important to keep the doses of dopamine agonists as low as possible.

MPTP

1-Methyl-4-phenyl-1,2,3,6-tetrahydropyridine (MPTP) is a compound that was discovered in 1979 at the National Institutes of Health [22]. MPTP has been used as a model compound since it kills dopaminergic neurons and produces the behavioral, neurochemical and pathological features of parkinsonism in man, monkeys, mice and possibly other species. Following the initial discovery of MPTP, extensive studies were made by Markey [23] and others [24] to investigate the mechanism of action. Chiba found that MPTP is oxidized by monoamine oxidase (MAO) to produce the neurotoxic agent, 1-methyl-4-phenylpyridine (MPP^+, 25). This is a four electron oxidation process. MPP^+ was found by Nicklas and others to be a weak and reversible inhibitor of complex 1 in mitochondria [26,27]. Of course, complex 1 inhibitors greatly impair energy production and increase the formation of oxygen radicals by mitochondria. However, MPP^+ must be concentrated to millimolar levels in mitochondria by an ATP requiring uptake mechanism before inhibition of complex 1 occurs. The inhibition of complex 1 results in the inhibition of ATP production in mitochondria and the subsequent release of MPP^+. Therefore, complex 1 inhibition is a self limiting mechanism with MPTP.

MPP^+ is a redox cycling agent, Figure (1). First a two electron reduction, hydride transfer, step occurs [28] with the production of 1-methyl-4-phenyl-1,4-dihydropyridine (DHP). DHP can then decay in one electron steps producing superoxide and peroxyl radical [29, 30]. DHP is unstable and either decomposes to methylamine and other products or is oxidized by superoxide to produce MPP radical. The formation of MPP radical is significant since it is a very strong reducing agent that can catalyze the formation of hydroxyl radical from hydrogen peroxide.

Direct, one electron reduction of MPP^+ is not possible in dopaminergic neurons since the reduction potential is about –1 V. Two electron reduction of MPP^+ by hydride transfer (H^-) is catalyzed by a number of enzymes, especially flavo enzymes, Figure (2). The hydride transfer process is thermodynamically favorable. Enzymes that can perform the hydride transfer include aldehyde dehydrogenase [30], xanthine oxidase [30], lipoamide dehydrogenase [30], mitochondrial complex 1 [31], cytochrome P450 reductase [32] and tyrosine hydroxylase [33]. Of course, NO synthase has cytochrome P450 reductase activity. Dopaminergic neurons are known to exhibit high cytochrome P450 reductase/NO synthase activity. Perhaps NO synthase can also catalyze the two electron reduction of MPP^+.

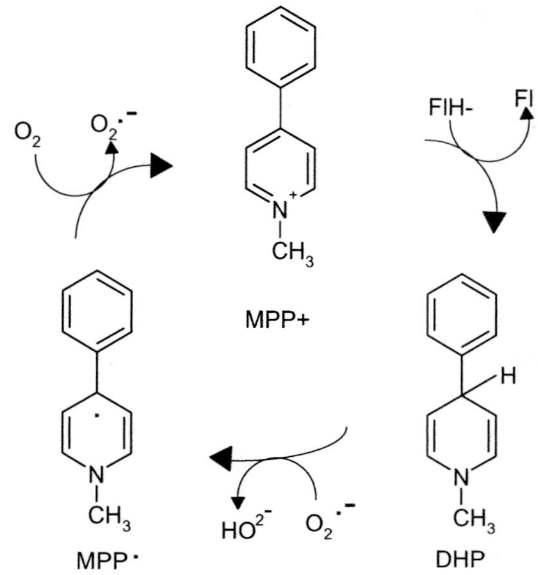

Figure 1. Mechanism of enzymatic reduction of MPP^+. This figure comes from reference 30 and is used with permission from Pergamon Press.

1) $MPP^+ + H^- \rightarrow DHP \quad E = 0.8\ V$

2) $DHP + O_2^{\cdot -} \rightarrow MPP^{\cdot} + OOH^{\cdot} \quad E = 2.8\ V$

3) $MPP^{\cdot} + O_2 \rightarrow MPP^+ + O_2^{\cdot -} \quad E = 0.9\ V$

4) $MPP^{\cdot} + H_2O_2 \rightarrow MPP^+ + HO^{\cdot} + HO^- \quad E = 1.6\ V$

Figure 2. Thermodynamics of MPP radical formation through hydride transfer and degradation by one electron oxidation.

Flavin in FAD bound to an enzyme can be reduced to an anionic semiquinone form. The anionic, reduced flavin readily binds MPP^+. The anionic semiquinone flavin reduces MPP^+ through hydride transfer. Xanthine oxidase and xanthine dehydrogenase are both flavo enzymes and are known to produce superoxide and hydrogen peroxide. Lipoamide dehydrogenase is a mitochondrial flavo enzyme that produces acetyl CoA from pyruvate. Complex 1 is an NADH dehydrogenase that contains flavin and iron. Cytochrome P450 reductase is a flavo enzyme.

1-Methyl-4-phenyl-2,3-dihydropyridine ($MPDP^+$) is a metabolite of MPTP. Trevor proposed that $MPDP^+$ is oxidized by MAO, a flavo enzyme, in one electron steps to produce MPP radical [34]. Incubation of MAO with $MPDP^+$ results in hydrogen peroxide, superoxide and perhaps hydroxyl radical [31]. This was the first evidence that MAO can produce oxygen radicals. MAO oxidizes MPTP to $MPDP^+$ and then to MPP radical.

Redox cycling of MPP^+ is a critical component of MPTP toxicity. MPTP crosses the blood brain barrier. It is oxidized by MAO B in glial and endothelial cells to produce MPP^+. Dopaminergic neurons contain MAO A. MAO B is required for the bioactivation of MPTP [35]. MPP^+ is toxic to endothelial and glial cells [36,37], that may rupture due to MPP^+ toxicity. This necrotic rupture releases MPP^+ into the extracellular fluids, where it is taken up by dopaminergic neurons in a process that competes with dopamine uptake [38]. In the neurons, MPP^+ redox cycles and weakly inhibits complex 1. This results in oxygen radical formation that causes DNA to fragment leading to necrosis and apoptosis [39].

Nicotinamide

Protection of DNA in dopaminergic neurons is an approach to the treatment of Parkinson's Disease that has not been considered previously. Nicotinamide, a vitamin B_3, has been shown to protect DNA in the midbrain during MPTP toxicity and decrease cell death [39]. Nicotinamide is a precursor for brain NAD. It is taken up rapidly into the brain and results in 50% increases in brain NAD levels within a few hours [40]. Niacin, another form of vitamin B_3, on the other hand, is not readily taken up into the brain. NAD is a substrate for poly(ADP-ribose) polymerase (PARP), a critical enzyme in DNA protection. PARP is activated by DNA nicks and double strand breaks. The enzyme binds to the ends of the nicked DNA and stabilizes them until repair can occur. PARP uses NAD to poly(ADP-ribosylate) several nuclear enzymes involved in DNA repair. This ribosylation process activates several repair enzymes and results in rapid restoration of DNA. However, the consequence of PARP activity is that NAD levels decrease [40]. NAD is an adenine containing compound. Depletion of NAD also leads to ATP depletion [41]. This loss of cellular energy compounds can be critical to the cell and may lead to cell death. Nicotinamide is a precursor for NAD and protects cellular NAD and ATP levels during oxidative stress [41].

As many as 30% of elderly people may be deficient in nicotinamide [42]. Of course, severe nicotinamide deficiency can lead to fatal neurodegeneration, known as Pellagra. However, the consequences of less severe nicotinamide deficiency are not known. Clinical trials have shown that NAD therapy is helpful in Alzheimer's disease and Parkinson's disease [43,44]. NAD is broken down in the gut to nicotinamide such that NAD is a delivery form for nicotinamide. Perhaps nicotinamide itself should be tested in Parkinson's disease to see if it slows down the progression of the disease.

What is the toxicity of nicotinamide? Niacin induces facial flushing, pruritis, hypotension, peptic ulcers, hyperglycemia, cardiac arrhythmias and can lower blood triglycerides. Nicotinamide is associated with none of these reactions. Nicotinamide can produce vasodilatation, induction of several enzymes and inhibition of the synthesis of other enzymes [45]. The major metabolic product of nicotinamide is NAD. A minor metabolite of nicotinamide is N-methylnicotinamide [45]. N-methylnicotinamide interacts with complex 1 in mitochondria to produce oxygen radicals and destroy complex 1 [46]. Injection of N-methylnicotinamide into the midbrain results in decreased dopamine in the striatum [46]. It is not clear how much N-methylnicotinamide is present in the brains of patients with Parkinson's disease. However, it may be important to use as low a dose as possible of nicotinamide in Parkinson's disease patients. Alternatively, N-methyltransferase inhibitors could be used to decrease N-methylnicotinamide formation.

Nicotinamide in excess can shorten the life span of some cells possibly by inhibiting Sir2 enzymes [47]. Calorie restriction is well known to extend life span. Calorie restriction may involve a certain amount of nicotinamide deficiency. Nicotinamide deficiency activates Sir2. PNC1 expression leads to the expression of nicotinamidase that converts nicotinamide into niacin, thereby causing nicotinamide deficiency. PNC1 is activated by calorie restriction. This is another line of evidence that suggests that nicotinamide must be used in low doses in Parkinson's disease.

Dopamine Oxidation by MAO

Dopamine can oxidize producing quinones, semiquinones and neuromelanin as mentioned previously. Presynaptic nerve terminals capture most of the dopamine released into the synapse and store it in vesicles to be reutilized. However, some dopamine does not reach the vesicles but instead encounters mitochondria where it may be metabolized by MAO B and MAO A to produce hydrogen peroxide, superoxide and hydroxyl radical [31]. MAO oxidation of dopamine results in an increase in hydrogen peroxide, which is detoxified by glutathione peroxidase with glutathione oxidation, a sign of oxidative stress induction in neurons [48]. Dopamine is oxidized by MAO to produce 3,4-dihydroxyphenylacetaldehyde. MAO is found in all mitochondria. The enzyme derives reducing equivalents from its substrates, typically amines. One electron is removed from the substrate to make the anionic semiquinone flavin. Dopamine is converted into an aminium radical cation that abstracts hydrogen from an adjacent carbon forming an imminium radical after loss of a proton, Figure (3). The imminium radical hydrolyzes to form an aldehyde and ammonia. The anionic semiquinone flavin can interact with oxygen to make hydrogen peroxide or oxygen radicals.

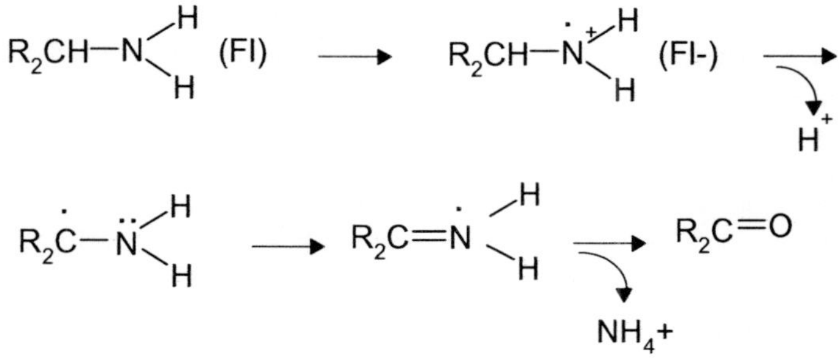

Figure 3. Monoamine oxidase mechanism.

In Parkinson's disease patients the neuronal levels of dopamine are low in the striatum. As dopamine levels decrease, the formation of oxygen radicals may also decrease. However, the turnover of dopamine may increase during the disease process [49] and during levodopa treatment such that oxygen radical formation may be high in some neurons. Levodopa, a dopamine precursor, is used to partly correct nigrostriatal dopamine deficiency.

Selegiline is an inhibitor or MAO B that is used in Parkinson's disease. Theoretically, inhibition of MAO B could decrease oxygen radical formation in the midbrain and could be neuroprotective. Is there any evidence that selegiline can slow down the progression of Parkinson's disease? The DATATOP study and studies by the Norwegian-Danish Study Group and the Swedish Parkinson Study Group found that selegiline can delay the need for levodopa therapy and slow down disease progression [50,51,52]. However, therapy with selegiline is problematic with postural hypotension, arrhythmias, hypertension and the serotonin syndrome decreasing the usefulness of the drug [53]. It interacts with fluoxetine, meperidine and other serotonin reuptake inhibitors to cause death or serious complications due to the serotonin syndrome [19]. Selegiline is an irreversible inhibitor of MAO B. This means that MAO B inhibition can only be corrected by synthesis of new MAO B. This is a process that may take 40 days [54]. Therefore, it makes no sense to use selegiline more than once every month. More frequent use of selegiline will result in overdosing and potential toxicity.

Aldehyde Dehydrogenase

Aldehyde dehydrogenase is composed of a diverse family of related enzymes involved in the oxidation of exogenous and endogenous aldehydes. It is fairly abundant in the brain. In the striatum, the majority of the enzyme is mitochondrial. Aldehyde dehydrogenase does not contain flavin. The enzyme interacts with aldehydes such as 3,4-dihydroxyphenylacetaldhyde (DOPAL) to produce 3,4-dihydroxyphenylacetic acid (DOPAC). Acids are produced from the reaction of aldehyde dehydrogenase and aldehydes. Complex I activity results in the oxidation of NADH to NAD. NAD is used by aldehyde dehydrogenase in the oxidation of DOPAL with the formation of NADH.

Mitochondrial (class 2, ALDH2) and cytosolic (class1, ALDH1) forms of human aldehyde dehydrogenase have been identified and characterized. They have 70% identity in their primary sequences. The distributions of human and rat aldehyde dehydrogenases are different in that human ALDH2 and ALDH1 are expressed in the brain at the same levels whereas in rat ALDH2 is the major enzyme.

The catalytic center of aldehyde dehydrogenase contains a sulfhydryl and NAD^+. The sulfhydryl may exist as a thiolate anion under some conditions. The aldehyde binds to the sulfhydryl, Figure (4). This allows NAD^+ to abstract hydrogen from the aldehyde forming a pyridinyl radical [55]. The sulfhydryl group stabilizes the substrate radical through double bond formation. An electron is then transferred to the pyridinyl radical forming NADH. The stability of the sulfhydryl radical may allow oxygen to interact forming superoxide. A second oxygen molecule may then interact with the pyridinyl radical forming more superoxide. Pyridinyl radical is more stable than a sulfur radical, which may explain the transfer of the radical from the sulfur to the pyridinyl moiety.

Of course, as mentioned above, aldehyde dehydrogenase can also perform hydride transfers. It may be that the majority of the catalytic mechanism occurs through a hydride transfer [56] from the substrate to NAD^+. This forms the sulfhydryl bound ketone that hydrolyzes making the product acid.

The structure of aldehyde dehydrogenase has been published [57]. The enzyme contains three domains, a catalytic domain, an NAD^+ binding domain, and a bridging domain. The domains interface at a 15 A long passage, shaped like a funnel, which leads to the catalytic pocket. NAD^+ binds to the enzyme in a novel mode, that is termed beta-alpha, beta mode. Perhaps this novel binding mode is responsible for the ability of the enzyme to perform single electron and two electron processes.

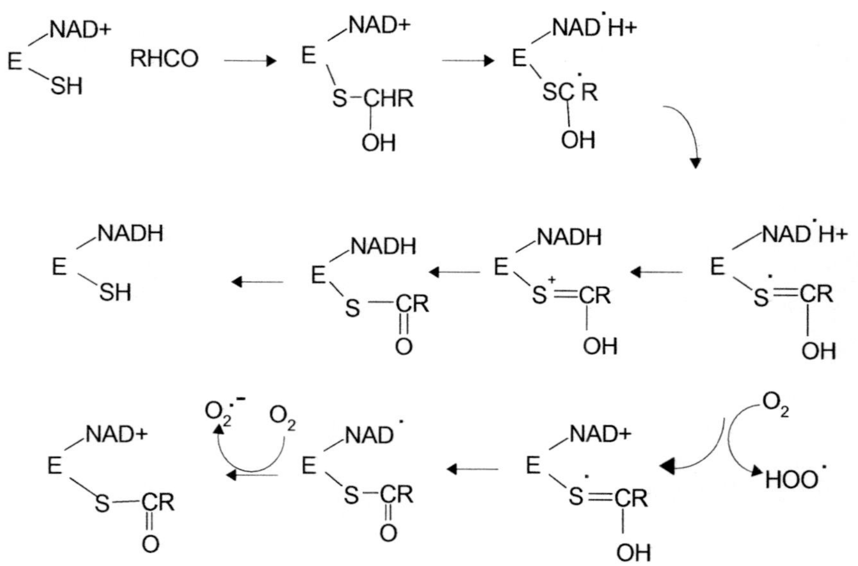

Figure 4. Aldehyde dehydrogenase mechanism. This figure comes from reference 52 and is used with permission from Pergamon Press.

Aldehyde dehydrogenase inhibitors are not used in Parkinson's disease. There is a mechanistic basis for aldehyde dehydrogenase inhibitors to slow down the progression of the disease, since they might inhibit oxygen radical formation. However, aldehyde dehydrogenase inhibitors have a serious interaction with ethanol. When a patient on an aldehyde dehydrogenase inhibitor drinks ethanol, severe nausea and vomiting can occur. This interaction would seriously limit the use of aldehyde dehydrogenase inhibitors in Parkinson's disease.

TYROSINE HYDROXYLASE

Tyrosine hydroxylase is the rate limiting enzyme in the synthesis of dopamine from tyrosine. The enzyme is uniquely found in dopaminergic and catecholaminergic neurons and adrenal cells. It contains iron and is a biopterin enzyme, not a flavo enzyme. The biopterin involved is (6R,6S)-5,6,7,8-tetrahydrobiopterin. Tyrosine hydroxylase activity decreases with aging due to increased deactivation [58]. The enzyme exists in 4 forms with TH1 and TH2 being the most abundant in the human brain [59]. Dopamine exerts feedback inhibition on the enzyme by binding to a specific site in the N-terminus [60]. As dopamine levels decrease in Parkinson's Disease, the feedback inhibition is released increasing oxygen radical formation by tyrosine hydroxylase. Levodopa increases dopamine levels in neurons reestablishing the feedback inhibition and decreasing oxygen radical formation. Therefore, rather than dopamine oxidation as the critical factor in oxygen radical formation, it appears that dopamine inhibition of tyrosine hydroxylase is a critical mechanism in decreasing oxygen radical formation Parkinson's Disease.

Tyrosine hydroxylase performs both two electron and one electron reductions. The primary catalytic mechanism involves one electron processes that result in 4a-carbinolamine *6* formation from tetrahydrobiopterin [33]. The two electron process is involved in the formation of tetrahydrobiopterin hydroperoxide *3* through hydride transfer. Of course tetrahydrobiopterin hydroperoxide can decompose forming the quinonoid dihydrobiopterin *4*.

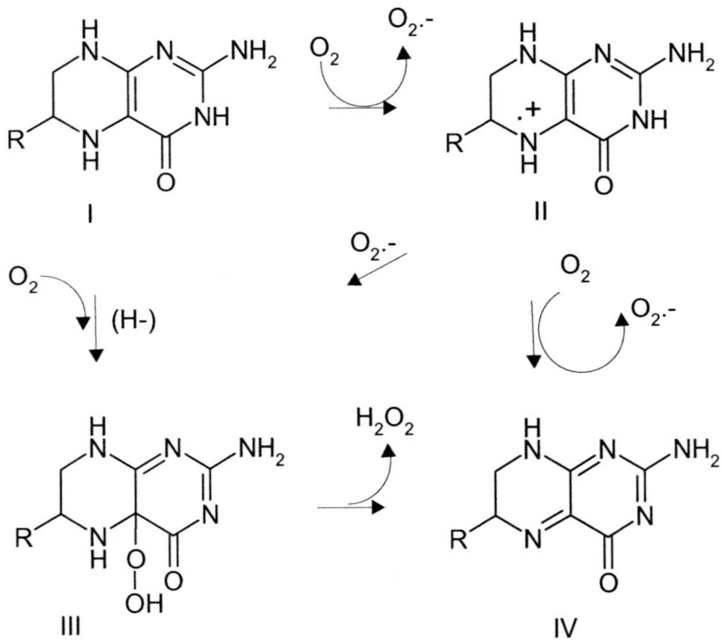

Figure 5. Mechanism of autoxidation of tetrahydrobiopterin. This figure comes from reference 33 and is used with permission from Maney Publishing.

Tetrahydrobiopterin can autoxidize, Figure (5), although this is of minimal importance *in vivo* since the free levels of tetrahydrobiopterin are very low. Tetrahydrobiopterin rearranges in solution forming pyrazino-s-triazine and imidazolones that react with tetrahydrobiopterin producing a radical cation *2*. In addition, a comproportionation reaction occurs between tetrahydrobiopterin and the quinonoid dihydrobiopterin producing the radical cation *2*. These reactions overcome the spin restriction between the reaction of triplet oxygen with singlet tetrahydrobiopterin. In addition, iron in the active site of tyrosine hydroxylase can catalyze the reaction and relieve the spin restriction. Finally, singlet oxygen is a dienophile and can react with tetrahydrobiopterin to produce tetrahydrobiopterin peroxide *3*, especially when catalyzed by a hydride transfer process. Hydride is donated by another tetrahydrobiopterin molecule.

Tyrosine hydroxylase proceeds through electron donation from tetrahydrobiopterin to ferric iron making the radical cation *2* without spin restriction, Figure (6). Iron does not have a spin restriction in this reaction since it has many valence states and outer shell electrons that give it some radical nature. The radical cation chelates iron making a stable complex. Oxygen can interact with the radical cation making an unstable intermediate similar to a peroxyl radical *7* or radical hydroperoxide *8*. The intermediate reacts with iron making the 4a-carbinolamine *6* and an active iron species that performs oxygen insertion reactions. The nature of this active iron species is unknown but may be iron(V) oxide. Alternatively, oxygen can interact with *2* to produce superoxide. Of course, there are other possible reactions of the unstable intermediates as demonstrated in Figure (7). Iron in the active site can cleave peroxide intermediates forming alkoxyl radicals. These radicals decompose by hydrogen abstraction reactions forming free radicals.

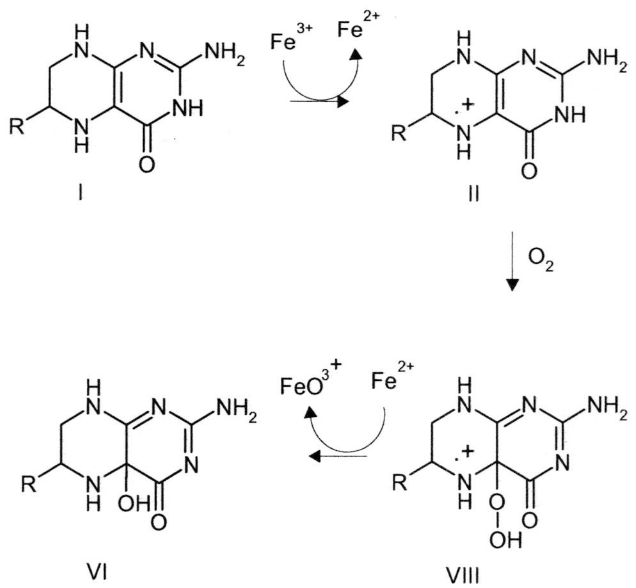

Figure 6. Catalytic mechanism of tyrosine hydroxylase. This figure comes from reference 33 and is used with permission from Maney Publishing.

The driving force in the reactions described is the oxidation of tetrahydrobiopterin. The one and two electron reduction potentials for tetrahydrobiopterin are 300 mV and 106 mV, respectively [61]. This is adequate for the one electron reduction of ferric iron (E_o' = 770 mV). The radical cation of tetrahydrobiopterin can reduce hydrogen peroxide making hydroxyl radical (H_2O_2 E_o' = 460 mV).

Other work has found similar results in terms of oxygen radical generation from tyrosine hydroxylase [62]. In fact, interaction of tyrosine hydroxylase with catechol quinones, such as dopamine quinones, may increase the formation of oxygen radicals by the enzyme [63]. This may involve the modification of sulfhydryls in the enzyme forming cysteinyl-catechols. A publication of the crystal structure of tyrosine hydroxylase [64] has shown that oxygen can form a bridge between iron and tetrahydrobiopterin, facilitating formation of tetrahydrobiopterin hydroperoxide.

Levodopa remains the mainstay of Parkinson's disease therapy [13]. Levodopa has two main mechanisms of action. First, it is a precursor for dopamine and can increase dopamine levels in the brain [65]. Second, by increasing dopamine levels it inhibits tyrosine hydroxylase and decreases oxygen radical formation [33]. Therapeutic levels of levodopa are adequate to fully inhibit tyrosine hydroxylase. Inhibition of tyrosine hydroxylase by dopamine decreases oxygen radical formation by the enzyme [33]. This is a neuroprotective effect. It is a mistake to call levodopa simply dopamine replacement therapy. Levodopa is the only agent known to prolong the lives of patients [9,10,11]. Prior to levodopa, patients usually died within 10 -15 years of diagnosis. Since levodopa, patients lead much longer lives. Levodopa is also much more effective against disease symptoms than any other agent [13,21].

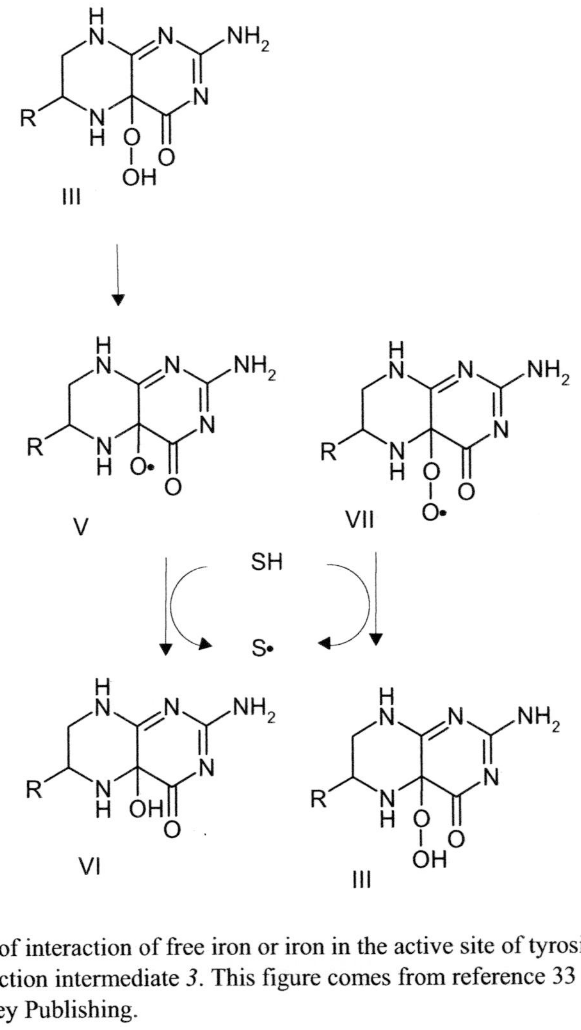

Figure 7. Mechanism of interaction of free iron or iron in the active site of tyrosine hydroxylase with the hydroperoxide reaction intermediate *3*. This figure comes from reference 33 and is used with permission from Maney Publishing.

Levodopa is clearly toxic *in vitro* to neurons [66]. Apparently, levodopa can nonenzymatically oxidize leading to oxygen radical formation [66]. This could lead to the involuntary movements (dyskinesias) and on-off phenomena (motor fluctuations) noted with levodopa, typically after 5 years or more of treatment. However, several studies have demonstrated clearly that disease duration correlates with dyskinesias and motor fluctuations, not duration of levodopa therapy, as recently reviewed [18]. This means that disease progression, not levodopa therapy, may be responsible for dyskinesias and motor fluctuations. Nonetheless, it is widely accepted that decreasing the dose of levodopa is a goal in Parkinson's disease. This can be done with dopamine agonists, selegiline and other agents.

There remains a need to test inhibitors of tyrosine hydroxylase, other than levodopa, in Parkinson's disease. Clearly, patients on levodopa exist for years with inhibited tyrosine hydroxylase. Can other inhibitors be used that do not oxidize nonenzymatically with oxygen radical formation? Tyrosine hydroxylase inhibitors in combination with a dopamine agonist or low dose levodopa could provide a new approach to the treatment of Parkinson's disease.

Conclusion

There are many mechanisms of oxygen radical formation in dopaminergic neurons. None of these mechanisms should be ignored. MAO induced oxygen radical formation may be important in Parkinson's disease. MAO B inhibition is already established therapy in Parkinson's disease, although the benefits to the patient may be mild. Administration of MAO A inhibitors can be very dangerous to patients given the food and drug interactions and the interaction with levodopa that can be life threatening. The possible formation of oxygen radicals by aldehyde dehydrogenase presents another difficult therapeutic problem. Inhibition of aldehyde dehydrogenase can produce very unpleasant reactions in patients who drink alcohol. Tyrosine hydroxylase induced oxygen radical formation may be very important in Parkinson's disease. The administration of levodopa causes dopamine levels to increase in dopaminergic neurons. This dopamine can inhibit tyrosine hydroxylase through feed back inhibition. Therefore, the inhibition of tyrosine hydroxylase is already a mainstay of Parkinson's disease therapy. Nicotinamide protects neuronal DNA, is neuroprotective and has yet to be explored as a means of slowing down the progression of Parkinson's Disease.

Recently, several studies and the American College of Neurology have recommended starting therapy with dopamine agonists. However, without studies that clearly show a prolongation of lifespan in patients treated with dopamine agonists, it is unwise to abandon levodopa. Levodopa must remain the first line of defense in Parkinson's disease until something else is clearly shown to prolong the lives of patients. The levodopa dose can be kept low and still fully inhibit tyrosine hydroxylase. Low dose dopamine agonists or other agents can be added to provide effective therapy.

References

[1] Adams, J. D. Agents used in neurodegenerative disorders. In: *Burger's Medicinal Chemistry and Drug Discovery, volume3,* ME Wolff, ed. John Wiley and Sons, New York, 1996, pp 261-319.

[2] Adams, J. D. Antiparkinsonian drug therapy. *Am. J. Pharmac. Ed.*, 1991, 55, 173-176.

[3] Adams, J. D., Mukherjee, S. K., Klaidman, L. K., Chang, M. L., Yasharel, R. Apoptosis and oxidative stress in the aging brain. *Ann. NY Acad. Sci.* 1996, 786, 135-151.

[4] Hoffmann, S., Spitovsky, D., Radicella J. P., Epe, B., Wiesner, R. J. Reactive oxygen species derived from the mitochondrial respiratory chain are not responsible for the basal levels of oxidative base modifications observed in nuclear DNA of mammalian cells. *Free Rad. Biol. Med.* 2004, 36, 765-773.

[5] Adams, J. D., Odunze, I. N. Oxygen free radicals and Parkinson's disease. Free Radic. *Biol. Med.*, 1991, 10, 161-169.

[6] Graham, D. G. On the origin and significance of neuromelanin. *Arch. Path. Lab. Med.*, 1979,103, 359-362.

[7] Graham, D. G., Tiffany, S. M., Bell, W. R., Gutknecht, W. F. Autoxidation versus covalent binding of quinones as the mechanism of toxicity of dopamine, 6-hydroxydopamine, and related compounds toward C1300 neuroblastoma cells in vitro. Mol. *Pharmacol.*, 1978, 14, 644-653.

[8] Mann, D. M. A., Yates, P. O. Pathogenesis of Parkinson's disease. *Arch. Neurol.*, 1982, 39, 545-549.

[9] Hoehn, M. M., Yahr, M. D. Parkinsonism: onset, progression and mortality. *Neurol.* 1967, 17, 427-42.

[10] Zumstein, H., Siegfried J. Mortality among Parkinson patients treated with L-dopa combined with a decarboxylase inhibitor. *Eur. Neurol.* 1976, 14, 321-8.

[11] Uitti, R. J., Ahlskog, J. E., Maraganore, D. M., Muenter, M. D., Atkinson, E. J., Cha, R. H., O'Brien, P. C. Levodopa therapy and survival in idiopathic Parkinson's disease: Olmstead county project. *Neurol.* 1993, 43, 1918-26.

[12] Parkinson Study Group. Safety and efficacy of pramipexole in early Parkinson's disease. A randomized dose ranging study. *JAMA* 1997, 278, 125-30.

[13] Clarke, C. E., Guttman, M. Dopamine agonist monotherapy in Parkinson's disease. *Lancet* 2002, 360, 1767-9.

[14] Gerlach, M., Double, K., Reichmann, H., Riederer, P. Arguments for the use of dopamine receptor agonists in clinical and preclinical Parkinson's disease. *J. Neural Transm. Supp.* 2003, 65, 167-83.

[15] Parkinson Study Group. Dopamine transporter brain imaging to assess the effects of pramipexole vs levodopa on Parkinson Disease progression. *JAMA* 2002, 287, 1653-61.

[16] Rakshi, J. S., Pavese, N., Uema, T., Ito, K., Morrish, P. K., Bailey, D. L., Brooks, D. J. A comparison of the progression of early Parkinson's disease in patients started on ropinirole or L-dopa: an ^{18}F-dopa PET study. *J. Neural Transm.* 2002, 109, 1433-1443.

[17] Whone, A. L., Watts, R. L., Stoessl, A. J., Davis, M., Reske, S., Nahmias, C., Lang, A. E., Rascol, O., Ribeiro, M. J., Remy, P., Poewe, W. H., Hauser, R. A., Brooks, D. J.

Slower progression of Parkinson's disease with ropinirole versus levodopa: the REAL-PET study. *Ann. Neurol.* 2003, 54, 93-101.

[18] Ahlskog, J. E. Slowing Parkinson's disease progression. *Neurol.* 2003, 60, 381-9.

[19] Drug Facts and Comparisons, Facts and Comparisons, St. Louis, 2003.

[20] Ahlskog, J. E. Parkinson's disease: is the initial treatment established? Curr. *Neurol. Neurosci. Rep.* 2003, 3, 289-95.

[21] Lange, K. W. Clinical pharmacology of dopamine agonists in Parkinson's disease. *Drugs Aging* 1998, 13, 381-9.

[22] Davis, G. C., Williams, A. C., Markey, S. P., Ebert, M. H., Caine, E. D., Reichert, C. M., Kopin, I. J. Chronic parkinsonism secondary to intravenous injection of meperidine analogues. *Psychiat. Res.*, 1979, 1, 249-254.

[23] Johannessen, J. N., Adams, J. D., Schuller, H. M., Bacon, J. P., Markey, S. P. 1-Methyl-4-phenylpyridine induces oxidative stress in the rodent. *Life Sci.,* 1986, 38, 743-749.

[24] Langston, J. W., Ballard, P., Tetrud, J. W., Irwin, I. Chronic parkinsonism in humans due to a product of meperidine analog synthesis. *Science,* 1983, 219, 979-980.

[25] Chiba, K., Trevor, A. J., Castagnoli, N. Metabolism of the neurotoxic tertiary amine, MPTP, by brain monoamine oxidase. *Biochem. Biophys. Res. Commun.*, 1984, 120, 573-578.

[26] Nicklas, W. J., Youngster, S. K., Kindt, M. V., Heikkila, R. E. Molecular mechanisms of MPTP induced toxicity IV. MPTP, MPP+ and mitochondrial function. *Life Sci.,* 1987, 40, 721-729.

[27] Ramsay, R. R., Salach, J. I., Dadgar, J., Singer, T. P. Inhibition of mitochondrial NADH dehydrogenase by pyridine derivatives and its possible relation to experimental and idiopathic parkinsonism. *Biochem. Biophys. Res. Commun.*, 1986, 135, 269-275.

[28] Oturan, M. A., Dostert, P., Benedetti, M. S., Moiroux, J., Anne, A., Fleury, M. B. One electron and two electron reductions of MPP^+. *J. Electroanal. Chem.*, 1988, 242, 171-179.

[29] Adams, J. D., Klaidman, L. K., Cadenas, E. MPP^+ redox cycling: a new mechanism involving hydride transfer. *Ann. NY Acad. Sci.,* 1992, 648, 239-240.

[30] Klaidman, L. K., Adams, J. D., Leung, A. C., Kim, S. S., Cadenas, E. Redox cycling of MPP^+: evidence for a new mechanism involving hydride transfer with xanthine oxidase, aldehyde dehydrogenase and lipoamide dehydrogenase. *Free Radic. Biol. Med.*, 1993, 15, 169-179.

[31] Adams, J. D., Klaidman, L. K., Leung, A. C. MPP^+ and $MPDP^+$ induced oxygen radical formation with mitochondrial enzymes. *Free Radic. Biol. Med.*, 1993, 15, 181-186.

[32] Sinha, B. K., Singh, Y., Krishna, G. Formation of $O_2^{\cdot-}$ and $HO^{\cdot}$ From MPP^+: reduction and activation by NADPH cytochrome P450 reductase. *Biochem. Biophys. Res. Commun.*, 1986, 135, 583-588.

[33] Adams, J. D., Klaidman, L. K., Ribeiro, P. Tyrosine hydroxylase: mechanisms of oxygen radical formation. *Redox Rep.* 1997, 3, 273-279.

[34] Trevor, A. J., Castagnoli, N., Singer, T. P. The formation of reactive intermediates in the MAO catalyzed oxidation of the nigrostriatal toxin MPTP. *Tox.,* 1988, 49, 513-519.

[35] Grimsby, J., Toth, M., Chen, K., Kumazawa, T., Klaidman, L., Adams, J. D., Karoum, R., Gal, J., Shih, J. Mice lacking MAO B show marked increases in beta-phenylethylamine, stress responsiveness, and resistance to MPTP toxicity. *Nature Genet.*, 1997, 17, 206-210.

[36] Adams, J. D., Kalivas, P. W., Miller, C. M. The acute histopathology of MPTP in the mouse CNS. *Brain Res. Bull.*, 1989, 23, 1-17.

[37] Adams, J. D., Klaidman, L. K., Odunze, I. N., Johannessen, J. N. Effects of MPTP on the cerebrovasculature. *Int. J. Develop. Neurosci.*, 1991, 9, 155-159.

[38] Javitch, J. A., D'Amato, R. J., Strittmatter, S. M., Snyder, S. H. Parkinsonism inducing neurotoxin, N-methyl-4-phenyl-1,2,3,6-tetrahydropyridine: uptake of the metabolite N-methyl-4-phenylpyridine by dopamine neurons explains selective toxicity. *Proc. Natl. Acad. Sci. USA,* 1985, 82, 2173-2177.

[39] Mukherjee, S. K., Klaidman, L. K., Yasharel, R., Adams, J. D. Increased brain NAD prevents apoptosis in vivo. *Eur. J. Pharmacol.,* 1997, 330, 27-34.

[40] Klaidman, L. K., Mukherjee, S. K., Adams, J. D. Oxidative changes in brain pyridine nucleotides and neuroprotection using nicotinamide. *Biochim. Biophys. Acta* 2001, 1525, 136-48.

[41] Yang, J., Klaidman, L. K., Nalbandian, A., Oliver, J., Chang, M. L., Chan, P. H. Adams, J. D. The effects of nicotinamide on energy metabolism following transient focal cerebral ischemia in Wistar rats. *Neurosci. Lett.* 2002, 333, 91-4.

[42] Bianchetti, A., Rozzini, R., Carabellese, C., Zanetti, O., Trabucchi, M. Nutritional intake, socioeconomic conditions, and health status in a large elderly population. *J. Am. Geriatr. Soc.* 1990, 38, 521-6.

[43] Birkmayer, J. G. D. Coenzyme nicotinamide adenine dinucleotide new therapeutic approach for improving dementia of the Alzheimer type. *Ann. Clin. Lab. Sci.* 1996, 26, 1-9.

[44] Birkmayer, J. G. D., Vrecko, C., Volc, D., Birkmayer, W. Nicotinamide adenine dinucleotide a new therapeutic approach to Parkinson's disease. *Acta Neurol. Scand.* 1993, 87 (sup 146), 32-5.

[45] Adams, J. D., Klaidman, L. K., Morales, M., Moran, K., Schiavoni, B., Hsu, J. R., Mukherjee, S. K. *Nicotinamide and neuroprotection.* Chemicals and Neurodegenerative Diseases. Bondy, S. C., ed, Prominent Press, Scottsdale, 1999, pp. 231-262.

[46] Fukushima, T., Kaetsu, A., Lim, H., Moriyama, M. Possible role of 1-methylnicotinamide in the pathogenesis of Parkinson's disease. *Exp. Tox. Path.*, 2002, 53, 469-73.

[47] Yang, J., Klaidman, L. K., Adams, J. D. Update to medicinal chemistry of nicotinamide in the treatment of ischemia and reperfusion. *Med. Chem. Rev. Online*, in press.

[48] Cohen, G., Farooqui, R., Kesler, N. Parkinson's disease: a new link between monoamine oxidase and mitochondrial electron flow. *Proc. Natl. Acad. Sci. USA*, 1997, 94, 4890-4894.

[49] Adams, J. D. Parkinson's disease and oxygen free radicals. Neurol. Forum, 1993, 4, 2-14.

[50] Larsen, J. P., Boas, J., Erdal, J. E. Does selegiline modify the progression of early Parkinson's disease? Results from a five year study. The Norwegian-Danish Study Group. *Eur. J. Neurol.* 1999, 6, 539-47.

[51] Parkinson Study Group. Effects of tocopherol and deprenyl on the progression of disability in early Parkinson's disease. *NEJM* 1993, 328, 176-83.

[52] Palhagen, S., Heinonen, E. H., Hagglund, J., Kaugesaar, T., Kontants, H., Maki-Ikola, O., Palm, R., Turunen, J. Selegiline delays the onset of disability in de novo parkinsonian patients. Swedish Parkinson study group. *Neurol.* 1998, 51, 520-5.

[53] Anonymous. Selegiline: a second look. Six years later: too risky in Parkinson's disease. *Prescrire International* 2002, 11, 108-11.

[54] Fowler, J. S., Volkow, N. D., Logan, J., Wang, G. J., MacGregor, R. R., Schyler, D., Wolf, A. P., Pappas, N., Alexoff, D., Shea, C. Slow recovery of human brain MAO B after L-deprenyl (selegiline) withdrawal. *Synapse* 1994, 18, 86-93.

[55] Adams, J. D., Klaidman, L. K. Acrolein induced oxygen radical formation. *Free Radic. Biol. Med.*, 1993, 15, 187-193.

[56] Mann, C. J., Weiner, H. Differences in the roles of conserved glutamic acid residues in the active site of human class 3 and class 2 aldehyde dehydrogenase. *Protein Sci.*, 1999, 8, 1922-1929.

[57] Liu, Z. J., Sun, Y. J., Rose, J., Chung, Y. J., Hsiao, C. D., Chang, W. R., Kuo, I., Perozich, J., Lindahl, R., Hempel, J., Wang, B. C. The first structure of an aldehyde dehydrogenase reveals novel interactions between NAD and the Rossman fold. *Nature Struct. Biol.,* 1997, 4, 317-326.

[58] De La Cruz, C. P., Revilla, E., Venero, J. L., Ayala, A., Cano, J., Machado, A. Oxidative inactivation of tyrosine hydroxylase in substantia nigra of aged rat. *Free Radic. Biol. Med.*, 1996, 20, 53-61.

[59] Nagatsu, T. Genes for human catecholamine synthesizing enzymes. *Neurosci. Res.*, 1991, 12, 315-345.

[60] Nakashima, A., Mori, K., Suzuki, T., Kurita, H., Otani, M., Nagatsu, T., Ota, A. Dopamine inhibition of human tyrosine hydroxylase type 1 is controlled by the specific portion in the N-terminus of the enzyme. *J. Neurochem.*, 1999, 72, 2145-2153.

[61] Eberlein, G., Bruice, T. C., Lazarus, R. A., Henrie, R., Benkovic, S. J. The interconversion of the 5,6,7,8-tetrahydro, 7,8-dihydro and radical forms of 6,6,7,7-tetramethyldihydropterin. A model for the biopterin center of aromatic amino acid mixed function oxidases. *J. Am. Chem. Soc.*, 1984, 106, 7916-7924.

[62] Haavik, J., Almas, B., Flatmark, T. Generation of reactive oxygen species by tyrosine hydroxylase: possible contribution to the degeneration of dopaminergic neurons. *J. Neurochem.,* 1997, 68, 328-332.

[63] Kuhn, D. M., Arthur, R. E., Thomas, D. M., Elferink, L. A. Tyrosine hydroxylase is inactivated by catechol-quinones and converted to a redox-cycling quinoprotein: possible relevance to Parkinson's disease. *J. Neurochem.*, 1999, 73, 1309-1317.

[64] Goodwill, K. E., Sabatier, C., Stevens, R. C. Crystal structure of tyrosine hydroxylase with bound cofactor analogue and iron at 2.3 A resolution: self-hydroxylation of Phe300 and the pterin-binding site. *Biochem.*, 1998, 37, 13437-13445.

[65] Pletscher, A. Levodopa treatment of Parkinson's syndrome: past and future. *Adv. Neurol.* 1990, 53, 469-473.

[66] VonVoigtlander, P. F., Fici, G. J., Althaus, J. S. Pharmacological approaches to counter the toxicity of dopa. *Amino Acids* 1998, 14, 189-96.

In: Focus on Parkinson's Disease Research
Editor: Marianne J. Willow, pp. 97-107
ISBN 1-59454-924-9
© 2006 Nova Science Publishers, Inc.

Chapter VI

RESPIRATORY DYSFUNCTION AND PULMONARY REHABILITATION IN PATIENTS WITH PARKINSON'S DISEASE

Fusun Koseoglu* and Nılufer Kutay Ordu Gokkaya
Ankara Physical Medicine and Rehabilitation Education and Research Hospital, Cardio-Pulmonary Rehabilitation Unit, Ankara, Turkey

ABSTRACT

There is a group of neurological disorders that pulmonary principles can be applied. In this group, pulmonary dysfunction often complicates a variety of musculoskeletal, medical and central nervous system disorders, including travmatic brain injury, stroke, multiple sclerosis and Parkinson's Disease (PD).

Respiratory abnormalities have been noted in patients with PD since its initial description in 1817, and these respiratory problems commonly contribute to morbidity and mortality. A variety of respiratory problems such as aspiration pneumonia, respiratory dysrhytmias; whether or not associated with levodopa therapy, chronic or recurrent airflow limitation, acute respiratory failure and lung infection have been reported. Additionally, obstructive and restrictive ventilatory defects, upper-airway and intercostal muscle involvement have been documented in PD.

Different possible mechanisms such as involvement of the upper airway striated muscles, decreased arterial PO2, L-Dopa induced dyskinesias, systemic defect in mitochondrial function have been postulated to explain the respiratory dysfunction in PD.

The components of a pulmonary rehabilitation program include overall team assesment in a multidisciplinary fashion, breathing retraining, airway clearance tecniques, exercise training, patient education and smoking cessation, psychosocial intervention and follow-up.

* Correspondence concerning this article should be addressed to Dr. Fusun Koseoglu, Baris Sitesi, 53. Sokak, No:1, 06530, Bilkent, Ankara, Turkey. Phone: +90 312 285 50 60; Fax: +90 312 310 42 42; E-mail: tkoseoglu@yahoo.com.

The multidisciplinary pulmonary rehabilitation team consists of a physiatrist and a pulmonologist, respiratory, physical and occupational therapists, a psychiatrist or psychologist, a social worker, vocational counsellor, and a dietician.
Before entry to the rehabilitation program, measurements for assessing the pulmonary rehabilitation patient are pulmonary function testing, chest radiogram, quality of life indicators, oxygen saturation, and cardiopulmonary exercise testing.
Patients with PD with a variety of symptoms such as dyspnea on exertion, decreased exercise tolerance, difficulties during activities of daily living, mood changes, hypoxemia have been shown to benefit from pulmonary rehabilitation program.

Keywords: Parkinson's Disease, respiratory dysfunction, pulmonary rehabilitation

A Review of the Literature

Respiratory abnormalities reported in patients with Parkinson's Disease (PD) are associated with substantial morbidity and mortality [1,2,3,4,5]. Bronchial pneumonia and schock induced by pulmonary infection constitute the major cause of death and chocking is one of the main causes of aspiration pnuemonia [1,2,6]. The effects of PD on respiration are still debated. A variety of respiratory dysfunction have been described in association with PD. These include restrictive neuromuscular spirometric pattern, respiratory dysrhythmias, which may or may not be associated with L-dopa therapy, upper or lower airway obstruction , and diminished strength of the respiratory muscle [1,2,3,4,5,7,8,9,10,11,12,13,14,15,16].

Hovestadt et al. reported that PIF, PEF, FEF 50% and maximal static mouth pressure values were significantly below normal in patients with PD. Their results pointed to subclinical upper airway obstruction and decreased effective muscle strength in a significant proportion of patients [10].

Bogaard et al. determined that only the effort-dependent variables PEF and PIF significantly correlated with severity of the disease and decreased with increasing clinical disability. It has been concluded that a decreased or less coordinated respiratory muscle force was a major feature in the decreased peak flow and abnormal flow volume patterns [12].

Tzelepis et al. Demonstrated that patients with PD were able to perform single respiratory efforts well, but had difficulty performing repetetive inspiratory loaded ventilatory efforts. Pulmonary abnormalities have been explained by the global motor disability of these patients [13].

Many authors determined that the most common abnormality was an abnormal configuration of the flow volume loop in patients with PD [2,11,17]. Endoscopy of the upper airways of the patients showed either regular, rhytmic changes or irregular, jerky movements in the glottic and supraglottic structures. [2] (Fig1).

Reduced vocal cord abduction and adduction; abnormal vocal cord movement amplitude and mucosal waveform; laryngeal tremor and oropharyngeal dysfunction have been observed in patients with PD by laryngoendoscopy and barium swallow videoflouroscopy [18,19].

It has been suggested that the intrinsic laryngeal muscles surrounding the upper airway are almost invariably involved in the involuntary movement characteristic of the extrapyramidal disorders [2].

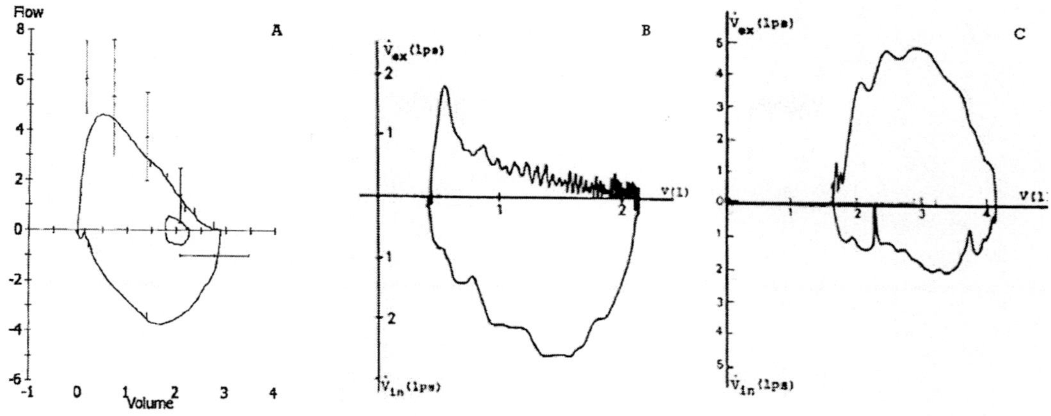

Figure 1. Panel A. Normal flow volume pattern Panel B. Patient with abnormal flow volume pattern (2) Panel C. Patient with abnormal flow volume pattern (2) Flow, Vex and Vin denote maximal expiratory and inspiratory flow rates, measured in liters Per second (lps). Volume and V denote volume (measured) in liters.

In a case report, Vincken showed that there was an improvement of parkinsonian and respiratory symptoms following oral administration of L-Dopa. This observation supported that extrapyramidal involvement of the striated upper airway musculature may limit airflow and cause respiratory symptoms [3].

EMG abnormalities of laryngeal muscles have been reported in patients with PD [2,3]. Probably the upper airway and its musculature have an automatic cyclic motor activity synchronized with the respiratory muscles. These structures also have other important tasks such as phonation, deglutition and protection of the lower respiratory tract. To accomplish all these activities it woul seem that a well-developed extrapyramidal control system is essential.

The diaphragm seems to be spared in extrapyramidal disorders. EMG of the respiratory muscles in patients with PD showed that the diaphragm exhibited a close to normal activity [1,2,3].Although diaphragmatic EMG was essentially normal, intercostal EMG demonstrated continued activity during expiration when these muscles normally are electrically quiet [4]. It has been proposed that cervical and dorsal arthrosis and kyphoscoliosis, seen in PD, could lead to a reduction of thorax and vertebral column mobilization, facilitating the development of pulmonary restriction [8]. This suggestion had been previously made by Senkman and Butler [20].

The high incidence of serious chest infections in patients with PD may be explained by a cough reflex impairment. The results of the Fontana's study indicated that reflex cough was impaired in patients with PD [21]. It is also likely that upper airway dysfunction is an important factor in retained secretions, atelectasis, aspirations and respiratory infections [2].

The medications used to treat these conditions can also produce respiratory disease. Dyskinesias involving the respiratory muscles have been described in a variety of movement disorders, especially tha tardive dyskinesia associated with long-term use of neuroleptic agents. Dyskinesias are a common complication of L-dopa therapy in idiopathic PD, occuring in 30 to 80 % of parkinsonian patients treated with L-dopa. It has been assumed that respiratory abnormality following L-dopa therapy may result from the choreiform movements or the rigidity-akinesia of respiratory muscle or from abnormal central control of ventilation [4,7,22]. These respiratory abnormalities appear after the introduction of L-dopa or an increase in L-dopa dose, and resolve with reduction of the dose or discontinuation of the drug. Rice et al postulated that alterations in dopaminergic receptor function in central respiratory circuits may conribute to L-dopa induced respiratory dyskinesias [22].

In contrast of these observations, many investigators showed that there was an improvement of respiratory dysfunction with L-dopa [14,23,24]. Breathing discomfort is attenuated after L-dopa intake [1,5]. Although this change of dyspnea is not related to changes in respiratory muscle performance or functions [5].

Patients with PD typically demonstrate slowness in initiating and performing movement as well as reduced excursion of movement. Overtime, Parkinsonian patients tend to adapt to these changes and gradually reduce the amount and variety of regular physical activity they perform, and become sedantary. The resultant chronic activity deconditions the muscles of locomotion. This in turn makes physical activity even more unpleasant and thus, reinforces the sedantary life style. Therefore, these patients do not report pulmonary symptoms.

It has been showed that there was a slight protective effect of physical exercise on the risk of developing PD [25,26]. On the other hand, a striking reduction in physical activity is found during the course of PD. Therefore, it has been suggested in previous investigations that exercise therapy is an important adjunt to the anti-parkinsonian medication [27,28,29,30].

Parkinsonian patients who were exercising exhibited the lowest mortality and increased life span [30,31]. Many studies reported that motor disability as well mood and subjective well-being could be clearly improved by exercise training program in early to medium stage PD patients [27,28,29,30,31,32]. However, it is not clear if the improvements are due to neurochemical alterations within the affected nigrostrial region or result from a more general efect of exercise on affect and motivation.

Chaouloff found an increse of dopamine release and turnover in rats during exercise and a decreased dopamine turnover after exercise due to a D2-receptor hypersensitivity in rats [33].

L-dopa pharmacokinetics and absorbtion might also be modified by exercise [34].

Tillerson et al proposed a combination of factors contributed to the dopamine sparing in mice forced exercise, including increased dopamine synthesis, turnover, and sprouting of surviving neuron terminals (plasticity of the remaining striatal dopamine system) [30].

It has been postulated that improvement in postural reflex and cortical reorganization especially in the supplemantary motor area might be a possible mechanism underlying the improvement by exercise [28].

Canning et al. determined that peak oxygen consumptions and peak work loads achieved by subjects with PD were not significantly different from normal values, despite evidence of respiratory and gait abnormalities typical of PD [35]. Exercise category significantly correlated with percent predicted VO2 peak, with sedantary subjects producing lower scores than exercising subjects. There was no significant correlation between disease severity and peak oxygen consumption. The results suggested that individuals with mild to moderate PD who perform regular aerobic exercise may maintain normal exercise capacity, despite the presence of typical abnormalities in respiratory function and gait. The authors emphasized that patients with PD should be encouraged to perform regular aerobic exercise to maintain exercise capacity and quality of life.

Sabate et al. investigated the effects of pulmonary dysfunction on activities of daily living (ADL) in patients with PD. Obstructive or restrictive pulmonary dysfunction and decreased arterial PO2 were observed in their parkinsonian patients in comparison with controls. They showed that PD patients with respiratory dysfunctions suffered greater deterioration in ADL than patients with normal pulmonary activity, although they had a smiliar degree of tremor, rigidity and bradykinesia. Thus, the results of this study suggested that the action of respiratory dysfunction on disability was not related to motor impairments . [8]

Although previous studies and clinical observations strongly suggest that incorporation of exercise in to a comprehensive treatment regimen for PD patients would be beneficial, it is difficult to develop a training program specific for motor disability improvement in PD. There are symptoms directly related to PD, functional problems that are due to aging process and additionally factors secondary to the disease like deconditioning and decreased endurance caused by impaired movements.

Concluding Remarks

Historically, pulmonary rehabilitation has been the cornerstone of the field of rehabilitation medicine. The roots of pulmonary rehabilitation extend back to the period when tuberculosis is quite prevalent before the 20th century [36]. Recently, The European Respiratory Society has provided the following definition: "Pulmonary rehabilitation is a process which systematically uses scientifically based diagnostic and treatment options to achieve the optimal daily functioning and health related quality of life of individual patients suffering from impairment and disability due to chronic respiratory disease as measured by clinically and/or physiologically relevant outcome measures." [37]. The multidisciplinary pulmonary rehabilitation team consist of physiatrists, internists, and pulmonologists, all of whom should be familiar with pulmonary disease, and therapists, nurses, nutritionists, social workers, case managers and psychologists.

Patients with COPD, restrictive lung disease, and sleep disordered breathing have been shown to benefit from pulmonary rehabilitation. Finally, there is a fourth clinical situation to which pulmonary rehabilitation principles can also be applied. In these clinical conditions, pulmonary dysfunction often complicates a variety of musculoskeletal, medical and central nervous system disorders, including traumatic brain injury, stroke, multiple sclerosis, and autoimmune deficiency syndrome. This situation has been little explored in the medical literature [38].

A variety of symptoms such as dyspnea on exertion, decreased exercise tolerance, difficulties during activities of daily living, mood changes, hypoxemia, weight changes, and soft tissue pain have been recognized for referral to pulmonary rehabilitation program [39].

The components of comprehensive pulmonary rehabilitation program include overall team assesment in a multidisciplinary fashion, education, breathing retraining, airway clearance techniques, supplemental oxygen therapy, exercise training, nutritional therapy and follow-up [37,40].

Before entry to the rehabilitation program, chest radiograph, pulmonary function testing (PFT), quality of life indicators, oxygen saturation, exercise testing are performed or measured in order to assess the pulmonary rehabilitation patient.

PFT makes it possible to evaluate future changes in pulmonary status and lung disease, and helps to determine possible impairments, and to identify whether a patient has a restrictive or obstructive pattern.

A baseline chest radiograph will help identify the possible coexistence of pulmonary pathology (e.g.,pneumonia or atelectasis).

Oxygen saturation, via oxygen pulse oximetry at rest and with exercise, may help to establish the need for oxygen supplementation.

Either General Health Questionnaires such as The Sickness Impact Profile (SIP) or Disease –Spesific Questionnaires such as Chronic respiratory Questionnaire can be used for the quantification of the impact of disease on daily life and well-being [41].

Exercise testing is very important for accurate measurement of exercise tolerance and to demonstrate changes overtime. Exercise testing for pulmonary rehabilitation can vary from a simple, timed walk measurement (e.g. six minute walk test) to complex incremental cardio-pulmonary exercise testing on a stationary bicycle, arm crank ergometer or treadmill. Exercise training is an essential feature of the pulmonary rehabilitation process [40,42]. Many of the effects of pulmonary rehablitation have been linked to the improvement of strength, endurance and the efficiency of the body's muscle function. Endurance training, upper extremity and ventilatory muscle strengtheninig, and breathing retraining can be used for exercise training.

Pursed lip breathing (PLB), air shifting and diaphragmatic breathing are the three major breathing retraining techniques that are used widely today. The goals of breathing retraing tecniques are:

1. To restore the diaphragm to a normal position and function,
2. To decrease the respiratory rate,
3. To diminish the work of breathing,
4. To reduce dyspnea and improve exercise performance [43,44].

PLB aims to improve expiration both by prolonging expiration and by preventing airway compression and airway collapse. PLB is a moderately active expiration through the half-opened lips inducing peak expiratory mouth pressures of about 5 cm H2O [44]. PLB reduces respiratory rate, dyspnea, and improves tidal volume and oxygen saturation [38,43,44].

Air shifting techniques involve taking a deep inspiration that is held with the glottis closed for 5 seconds, during which time the air shifts to lesser ventilated areas of the lungs. The subsequent expiration is via PLB. These techniques may be useful to decrease microatelectasis [38].

Diaphragmatic breathing aims to improve chest wall motion and ventilatation distribution, decrease energy cost of breathing, decrease the contribution of rib cage muscles, decrease dyspnea and improve exercise performance. To make this maneuver, the patient is told to move the abdominal wall exclusively during inspiration and reduce upper rib cage motion. Two studies observed a decrease in EMG activity of the sternomastoids and of the pectoralis major muscle during diaphragmatic breathing. Decreased respiratory rate and increased minute ventilation and tidal volume associated with improved blood gases were also reported after diaphragmatic breathing training [38,43,44].

The methods of ventilatory muscle training are voluntary isocapneic hyperpnea, inspiratory resistive loading and inspiratory threshold loading. Techniques of voluntary isocapneic hyperpnea provides low tension and high level of repetetive activity for the diaphragm and other inspiratory muscles. During inspiratory resistive breathing, the patient inspires through a mouth piece and adapter with an adjustable diameter. This resistance is flow-dependent. However, it became apparent that many of the subjects of inspiratory resistive training consciously or unconsciously reduced their inspiratory flow rates and lenghthened their inspiratory time to reduce the severity of the imposed loads [38]. More recently a flow-independent resitance device was developed. Threshold loading device has a valve that opens at acritical mouth pressure.

Ventilatory muscle training has been shown to improve exercise capacity more than exercise training alone, decrease dyspnea and nocturnal desaturation time and increase endurance capacity of ventilatory muscle [38,44,45,46].

Many neck, arm, and shoulder muscles are also accessory muscles of respiration. Thus, in patients with respiratory problems, these muscles participate both in breathing activities and in the positioning or moving of the upper chest and upper extremity for daily living activities. The overlap in function explains why patients with lung disease are particularly shorth of breath when performing upper extremity activities of daily living [37,47,48].

There are many types of upper extremity exercises such as arm crancking, simple anterior elevation of the arms, gravity resistance exercises, swimming and rowing. It has been shown that training of the arms in healthy subjects increases VO2 max, and decrease ventilatory requirement at identical work rates [47,48].

Many authors observed significant improvements in specific upper extremity performance tests after upper extremity training in comparison to control group [46,48,49].

Treadmill, upper and lower extremity ergometer can be used for endurance training. Endurance training involves a larger muscle mass working at moderate intensity for a longer period of time. This type of exercise is often carried out by starting with a comfortable exercise level for the pulmonary patient, which should allay the patient's fears of worsening is dyspnea and hypoxemia. Exercise intensity is gradually increased to maximal exercise as tolerated.

Exercise intensity can be described using target heart rate, maximum oxygen consumption, and the Borg rating of perceived exertion scale. This indicator is usually scored 0 to 10, with 0 indicating no discomfort or restlessness and 10 indicating extremely severe exertion or dyspnea.

The exercise sessions will often include at least 20 minutes (and preferably 30-60 minutes) of continuous activity. 3 to 5 days weekly exercise session frequency is the goal for the most pulmonary rehabilitation programs. The training program longer than 3 weeks (and preferably 5-10 week) is required to achieve a physiologic training effect. According to a recent meta-analysis, the minumum duration of rehabilitation programs is usually three months [50].

A recent review of 48 pulmonary rehabilitation studies indicated that consistent improvements included decreases in the ventilatory equivalent or the ventilation/oxygen consumption ratio, increases in work efficiency (external work per unit of oxygen consumed) and, thus, in exercise tolerance, ambulation capacity, generally well-being, dyspnea tolerance and quality of life measures [37,38].

Few studies have reported the effects of exercise training program on the respiratory dysfunction seen in patients with PD [5].

We investigated the effects of ventilatory and upper extremity muscle training and breathing retraining, as a part of comprehensive pulmonary rehabilitation program, on pulmonary function tests and exercise tolerance in patients with PD. Nine patients with PD participated in a 5 week exercise training program for one hour, three times Per week. Training program included diaphragmatic breathing, air shifting techniques, voluntary isocapneic hyperpnea and unsupported upper extremity exercise.

When compared with the healthy controls, the values of FVC, FEV1, FEF25-75%, MVV, PEF, PIF, VC and distance walked in six minutes were decreased in patients with PD. Many types of respiratory dysfunction such as spirometric restrictive ventilatory defect, generalized airway obstruction and abnormal flow-volume loop contour were determined in our patients.

We observed a slight improvement in flow volumes, lung volumes, ventilatory requirements (VE, VT, RR) for the same single respiratory effort and in ventilatory muscle force for the same repetetive respiratory maneuver after 5 week exercise training program. Also, there was a statistically significant increase in exercise tolerance and decrease in Borg RPE scale score at the end of the training program [17].

Although we did compare some values statistically, our findings suggested that exercise training can decrease ventilatory requirements for a given workload, increase ventilatory muscle force and exercise tolerance and improve the effort dependent spirometry variables and ventilatory pattern (larger VT, lower RR) during exercise.

The results from a small sample of PD patients are promising that exercise training, as a part of pulmonary rehabilitation program, may offer a potential therapeutic adjunct to current PD therapies in the future. Controlled studies in larger group of patients are required to determine the effects of pulmonary rehabilitation on respiratory limitations seen in PD.

Moreover, despite the presence of typical abnormalities in respiratory function, most PD patients do not report respiratory symptoms. Respiratory disorders might be more important in exercise tolerance for strenuous exercise than in activities of daily living. Therefore, the evaluation of respiratory dysfunction should be systematically included in the daily management of these patients.

REFERENCES

[1] Vercueill L, Linard JP, Wuyam B, Pollak P, Bencherit G. Breathing pattern in patients with Parkinson's Disase. *Respiratory Physiology* 1999; 163-172.

[2] Vincken WG, Gauthier SG, Dollfus RE, Hanson RE, Darauay CM, Cosio MG. Involvement of upper airway muscles in extrapyramidal disorders: a cause of airflow limitation. *N Eng J Med* 1984; 311: 438-442.

[3] Vincken WG, Darauay, CM, Cosio MG. Reversibility of upper airway obstruction after L-Dopa therapy in Parkinson's Disase. *Chest* 1989; 96: 210-212.

[4] Brown LK. Respiiratory dysfunction in Parkinson's Disase. *Clin Chest Med* 1994; 15: 715-727.

[5] Weiner P, Inzelberg R, Davidovich A, Nisipeanu P, Magadle R, Berar-Yanay N, Carasso R. Respiratory Muscle performance and the perception of dyspnea in Parkinson's Disase. *Can J Neurol Sci* 2002; 29: 68-72.

[6] Wang X, You C, Chen H, Caı X. Clinical course and cause of death in elderly patints with idiopathic Parkinson's Disase.. *Chin Med* 2002; 115(9): 1409-1411.

[7] Zupnick HM, Brown LK, Miller A, Moros DA. Respiratory dysfunction due to L-Dopa therapy for parkinsonism; diagnosis using serial pulmonary function tests and respiratory inductive plethysmography. *Am J Med* 1990; 89: 109-114.

[8] Sabate M, Rodriguez M, Mendez E, Enriguez E, Gonzalez I. Obstructive and restrictive pulmonary dysfunction increases disability in Parkinson's Disase. *Arch Phy Med Rehabil* 1996; 77: 29-34.

[9] Sabate M, Gonzales I, Ruperez F, Rodriguez M. Obstructive and restrictive pulmonary dysfunction in Parkinson's Disase. *J Neurol Sci;* 1996; 138: 114-119.

[10] Hovestadt A, Bogaard JM, Meerwaldt J, Van der Meche FG, Stigt J. Pulmonary function in Parkinson's Disase. *J Neurol Neyrosurg Psychiatry* 1989; 52: 329-333.

[11] Izquierrdo-Alanso JL, Jimenez- Jimenez FJ, Cabrera-Valdivia F, Mansilla- Lesmes M. Airway dysfunction in patients with Parkinson's Disase. *Lung* 1994; 172: 47-55.

[12] Bogaard JM, Hovestad A, Meerwaldt J, Van der Meche FGStigt J. Maximal expiratory and inspiratory flow-volume curves in Parkinson's Disase. *American Review of Respiratory Diseases* 1989; 139: 610-614.

[13] Tzelepis G, Mc Cool FD, Friedman JH. Respiratory muscle dysfunction in Parkinson's Disase. *American Review of Respiratory Diseases* 1988; 138: 266-271.

[14] Herer B, Arnulf I, Housset B. Effects of levodopa on pulmonary function in Parkinson's Disease. *Chest* 2001; 119-387-393.

[15] De Pandis MF, Starace A, Stefanelli F, Maruzzo P, Meoli I, De Simone G. Prati R, Stocchi F. Modification of respiratory function parameters in patients with severe Parkinson's Disase. *Neurol Sci* 2002; 23: 69-70.

[16] Polatli M, Akyol A, Cilda O, Bayulkem K. Pulmonary function tests in Parkinson's Disase. *Eur J Neurol* 2001; 8: 341.

[17] Koseoglu F, Inan L, Ozel S, Demir Deviren S, Karabiyikoglu G, Yorgancioglu R, Atasoy T, Ozturk A. The effects of a pulmonary rehabilitation program on pulmonary function tests and exercise tolerance in patients with Parkinson's Disase. *Funct Neurol* 1997; 12: 319-325.

[18] Stelzig Y, Hochhaus W, Gall V, Henneberg A. Laryngeal manifestations in patiensts with Parkinson's Disase. *Laryngo-Rhino-Otologie* 1999; 78: 544-551.

[19] Wintzen AR, Badrising UA, Roos RA, Vielvoye J, Liauw L, Pauwels EK. Dysphagia in ambulant patients with Parkinson's Disase: common, not dangerous. *Can J Neurol Sci* 1994; 21: 53-56.
[20] Schenkman M, Butler RB. A model for multisystem evaluation treatment of individuals with Parkinson's Disase. *Phys Ther* 1989; 69: 932-943.
[21] Fontana GA, Pantaleo T, Lavorini F, Benvenuti F, Gangemi S. Defective motor control of coughing in Parkinson's Disase. *Am J Respir Crit Care Med* 1998; 158: 458-464.
[22] Rice JE, Antic R, Thompson PD. Disordered respiration as a Levodopa- Induced Dyskinesia in Parkinson's Disease. *Movement Disorders* 2002; 17: 524-527.
[23] Nakane KK, Bass H, Tyler HR. Levodopa in PD. Arch Intern Med 1972; 130, 346-348.
[24] De Bruin VMS, Lees A. Effects of treatment on airway dynamics and respiratory muscle strength in Parkinson's Disase. *Am Rev Respir Dis* 1993; 148: 176-180.
[25] Brasted PJ, Watts C, torres EM, Robbins TW, Dunnett SB. Behavioural recovery following striatal transplantation: Effects of postoperative training and P-zone volume. *Exp Brain Res* 128: 535-538.
[26] Sasco AJ, Paffenbarger RS, Gendre I, Wing Al. The role of physical exercise in the occurence of PD. *Arch Neurol* 49; 360-365.
[27] De Goede CJT, Keus SHJ, Kwakkel G, Wagenaar RC. The effects of physical therapy in Parkinson's Disease: A research synthesis. *Arch Phys Med Rehabil* 2001; 82: 509-515.
[28] Miyai I, Fujimato Y, Ueda Y, Yamamato H, Nozaki S, Saito T, Kang J. Treadmill training with body weight support: Its effect on Parkinson's Disase. *Arch Phys Med Rehabil* 2000; 81: 849-852.
[29] Scandalis TA, Bosak A, Berliner JC, Helman LL, Wells MR. Resistance training and gait function in patients with Parkinson's Disase. *Am J Phys Med Rehabil* 2001; 80; 38-43.
[30] Tillerson JL, Caudle WM, Reveron ME, Miller GW. Exercise ınduces behavioral recovery and attenuates neurochemical deficits in rodent models of Parkinson's disease. *Neuroscience* 2003; 119: 899-911.
[31] Reuter I, Engelhardt M, Stecker K, Baas H. Therapeutic value of exercise training in Parkinson's disease. *Medicine & Science in Sports & Exercise* 1999: 1544-1549.
[32] Bergen JL, Toole T, Elliott RG, Wallace B, Robinson K, Maitland CG. Aerobic exercise intervention improves aerobic capacity and movement initiation in Parkinson's disease patients. *Neurorehabilitation* 2002; 17: 161-168.
[33] Chaouloff F. Physical exercise and brain monoamines: a review. *Acta Physiol Scand* 1989; 137: 1-13.
[34] Cartes JH, Nutt JG, Woodward WR. The effect of exercise on levodopa absorbtion. *Neurology* 1992; 42: 2042-2045.
[35] Canning CG, Alison JA, Allen NE, Groeller H. Parkinson's Disease: an investigation of exercise capacity, respiratory function, and gait. *Arch Phys Med rehabil* 1997; 78: 199-207.
[36] Pety TL. Pulmonary Rehabilitation: A personal historical perpective. In: *Casaburi R, Petty LT, eds. Principles and Practice of Pulmonary Rehabilitation*. Philadelphia: W.B. Saunders Company 1993; p:1-8.

[37] Clark CJ, Decramer M. The definition and rationale for pulmonary rehabilitation. In: Donner CF, Decramer M, eds. Pulmonary Rehabilitation. European Respiratory Monograph. UK: ERS Journals Ltd; 2000, p:1-6.

[38] Bach JR. Rehabilitation of the patient with respiratory dysfunction In: *De Lisa JA, Gans BM, eds. Rehabilitation Medicine*. Philadelphia; Lippincott-Raven Publishers 1998: 1359-1385.

[39] Goldstein RS, Avendeano MA. Candidate evaluation. In: *Casaburi R, Petty TL, eds. Principles and Practice of Pulmonary Rehabilitation*. Philadelphia: W.B. Saunders Company 1993; p:317-312.

[40] Glassman SJ. Pulmonary Dysfunction. In: *shankar K ed. Exercise Prescription*. Philadelphia; Hanley- Belfus Inc. 1998; p: 133-144.

[41] Carone M, Jones PW. Health status " quality of life "In: Donner CF, Decramer M, eds. Pulmonary Rehabilitation. *European Respiratory Monograph*. UK: *ERS Journals Ltd*; 2000, p: 22-35.

[42] Zuwallack RL. Outcome measures for pulmonary rehabilitation In: Donner CF, Decramer M, eds. Pulmonary Rehabilitation. *European Respiratory Monograph. UK: ERS Journals Ltd;* 2000, p: 177-198.

[43] Faling LS. Controlled breathing techniques and chest physical therapy in chronic obstructive pulmonary disease and allied conditions. In: *Casaburi R, Petty TL, eds. Principles and Practice of Pulmonary Rehabilitation*. Philadelphia: W.B. Saunders Company 1993; p: 167-183.

[44] Gosselink R, Houtmeyers E. Physiotherapy. In: Donner CF, Decramer M, eds. Pulmonary Rehabilitation. European Respiratory Monograph. *UK: ERS Journals Ltd*; 2000, p: 70-89.

[45] Belman MJ. Ventilatory muscle training and unloading. In: *Casaburi R, Petty TL, eds. Principles and Practice of Pulmonary Rehabilitation*. Philadelphia: W.B. Saunders Company 1993; p: 225-239.

[46] Ries AL. The importance of exercise in pulmonary rehabilitation *Clin Chest Med* 1994; 15: 327-336.

[47] Casaburi R. Exercise training in chronic obstructive lund disease. In: *Casaburi R, Petty TL, eds. Principles and Practice of Pulmonary Rehabilitation*. Philadelphia: W.B. Saunders Company 1993; p: 1077-1082.

[48] Bartolome RC. The clinical use of upper extremity exercise in pulmonary rehabilitation. *Clin Chest Med* 1994; 15: 327-336.

[49] Lake FR, henderdon K, Briffa T, Openshaw J, Musk AW. Upper limb and lower limb exercise training in patients with chronic airflow obstruction. *Chest* 1990; 97: 1077-1082.

[50] Donner CF, Lusuardi M. Selection of candidates and programmes. In: Donner CF, Decramer M, eds. Pulmonary Rehabilitation. *European Respiratory Monograph. UK: ERS Journals Ltd;* 2000, p: 132-142.

In: Focus on Parkinson's Disease Research
Editor: Marianne J. Willow, pp. 109-120

ISBN 1-59454-924-9
© 2006 Nova Science Publishers, Inc.

Chapter VII

Movement Disorders in 14 Patients with Cerebral Tuberculomas

Fernando Alarcón*

Department of Neurology, Eugenio Espejo Hospital, Quito, Ecuador

Abstract

Background

Patients with cerebral tuberculomas may present movement disorders that have rarely been described in the literature.

Methods

We selected patients with cerebral tuberculomas who developed involuntary abnormal movements. We determined their clinical characteristics, location of the lesions, follow-up, and pathophysiological implications.

Design

Descriptive observational prospective study.

* Correspondence concerning this article should be addressed to: Dr. Fernando Alarcón, Eugenio Espejo Hospital, Department of Neurology, P.O. Box 17-07-9515, Quito, Ecuador, South America, Phones: (593-2) 2221-202 / (593-2) 2503-296, Fax: (593-2) 2505-157, E-mail: alyosha@access.net.ec

Results

We report 14 patients with tuberculomas, who developed movement disorders. Twenty-four months after treatment was completed, we determined an outcome for these patients. Seven patients had chorea, 4 tremor, 2 dystonia, and 1 myoclonus. The average age of the patients with chorea was lower than that of patients with dystonia ($p < 0.04$) and tremor ($p < 0.02$). One patient with tuberculoma and AIDS died. The disease was more severe in the patients with chorea and dystonia. Chorea was especially correlated with thalamic tuberculomas and tremor with fronto-parietal granulomas. The 2 patients with dystonia had hydrocephalus and tuberculomas with thalamic and cerebellar location. In all patients, the abnormal movement lasted for less than 2 months.

Conclusions

Chorea is the most common movement disorder seen in patients with cerebral tuberculomas, and it appears in young patients. Chorea and dystonia correlated better with deep tuberculomas and tremor, with surface granulomas. Abnormal movements improved completely during the antituberculous treatment. The presence of an abnormal movement may be the first and most evident manifestation of a cerebral tuberculoma. Movement disorders are frequent in patients with cerebral tuberculomas. Various pathogenic mechanisms are involved in the development of movement disorders.

Keywords: cerebral tuberculomas, movement disorders, pathogenesis

Cerebral tuberculoma is a relatively frequent etiology among intracranial expansive lesions in developing countries [1, 2]. There may be unusual reports of movement disorders during the course of tuberculomas [3-5]. Chorea-ballismus, dystonia, myoclonus and tremor have all been described [3-11]. The pathogenic mechanisms that have been proposed include direct pressure effect, brain edema, and ischemia [11]. The age of the patients could be a predisposing factor for presentation with certain types of abnormal movement. The frequency, location, and type of movement disorder seen in tuberculomas over a 14-year period are reported.

Patients and Methods

We conducted a descriptive observational prospective study. Three hundred patients with tuberculosis of the central nervous system were admitted to the Neurology Department of the Eugenio Espejo Hospital between January 1989 and January 2003 and completed a standard protocol. Forty-seven had brain tuberculomas, and 14 of them developed involuntary abnormal movements (IAMs). A careful follow-up was conducted for more than 24 months.

The diagnosis of definite tuberculomas was based on surgery or autopsy confirmation or when the CSF mycobacterial culture/AFB stain was positive and the finding in the computerized tomography (CT scan) or magnetic resonance imaging (MRI) was compatible with tuberculomas. In patients who did not have bacteriological confirmation, the diagnosis was considered to be positive when the patients had CT scan or MRI images compatible with tuberculomas, with cerebrospinal fluid (CSF) findings consistent with meningeal inflammation compatible with tuberculous meningitis, or the enzyme-linked immunosorbent assay (ELISA) or adenosine deaminase activity (ADA) in the CSF, and at least two of the following were positive: the culture of Mycobacterium tuberculosis taken from another tissue or body fluid, Mantoux test, chest roentgenogram, basal enhancement on the CT or MRI, a history of tuberculosis, and a clinical response to antituberculous treatment.

In all patients, we established the time of evolution of the disease prior to admission to hospital, the severity of the disease, the time interval between start of treatment and onset of the abnormal movement, the evolution of the abnormal movement, and the outcome.

In all patients, we evaluated the severity of the disease in accordance with the modified scale of the British Medical Research Council for tuberculous meningitis [12-13]. Stage 1: no definite neurological symptoms on admission or in the history before admission without intracranial hypertension; Stage 2: sign of slight clouding of consciousness and/or focal neurological signs such as cranial nerve palsies or hemiparesis, with or without intracranial hypertension; Stage 3: moderate or severe clouding of consciousness, convulsions, intracranial hypertension, focal neurological signs such as hemiplegia and paraplegia.

The outcome of patients was evaluated 24 months after antituberculous treatment was finished in accordance with Smith's modified scale for tuberculous meningitis [12, 14]. Category 1 was comprised of patients who had fully recovered and without neurological deficit; Category 2 included patients with slight sequelae who needed no help for any activity; Category 3 consisted of patients with moderate sequelae who needed help for certain activities; and Category 4 was for patients with severe sequelae who had become completely dependent on others for their daily activities.

None of the patients had abnormal movements before tuberculomas, and none were receiving neuroleptic drugs or oral contraceptives or had a family history of IAMs. In all patients, a CT scan or MRI with and without contrast was carried out the first week after involuntary movements appeared. We determined the number and location of the tuberculomas and the ischemic lesions.

We defined four types of movement disorders in accordance with the previously established criteria: chorea, dystonia, tremor, and myoclonus [15-19]. We classified chorea and dystonia according to their distribution: focal (affecting a single part of the body), segmental (affecting two or more contiguous parts of the body), multifocal (affecting more than one part of the body), unilateral (affecting the ipsilateral arm and leg), and generalized. Myoclonus can be classified clinically according to its distribution: focal, multifocal, and generalized. We classified tremor according to its location and whether it was classified as predominantly at rest, postural, or kinetic. The type of dystonia was classified as spontaneous, intensified by action, mobile dystonic spasms causing repetitive dystonic posturing, and fixed. Chorea was classified as spontaneous, intensified by action, and with ballistic movements. Myoclonus can be classified clinically according to presentation: spontaneous, action, and stimulus-sensitive [19].

We performed statistical analyses using t-test and X^2 to compare age, sex, and clinical characteristics among groups with chorea, tremor, and dystonia. We used the analysis of variance to compare age, time of evolution of the disease prior to admission to hospital, the time interval between start of treatment and onset of the abnormal movement, and evolution of the abnormal movement, among the patients with chorea, tremor, and dystonia. The nominal level of statistical significance was set at 0.05.

RESULTS

The average age of the entire population with tuberculomas was 29.3±18.5, similar to the age of the patients with abnormal movements (Table 1), and there were more female than male patients ($p = 0.04$). The average age of the 14 patients (4 males, 10 females) was 29.6 ± 17.5 years (range from 9 to 79 years). Chorea was the most common movement disorder (50%), and the patients where it was present were younger (20.2 ± 10.9 years) than the patients with other IAMs ($p = 0.04$). Dystonic patients were 39 ± 3 years of age, and those with tremor 43.7 ± 21 years (Table 1).

The duration of pre-admission symptoms was longer in the patients with tremor (7.5 ± 0.8 weeks) ($p = 0.02$) than in the patients with chorea (7 ± 2.5 weeks), dystonia (3.5 ± 0.5 weeks), and myoclonus (2 weeks). The shortest time interval between admission and onset of IAMs was found in the choreatic patients (7.8 ± 4.7 days) ($p = 0.03$), and the longest interval was found in patients with tremor (36.2 ± 23.8 days). The patients with dystonia and the patient with myoclonus had a similar interval (15 days). In 2 patients with chorea, the abnormal movements started before the diagnosis of tuberculomas. The latest onset of an IAM was 60 days after diagnosis of tuberculomas in one patient with tremor. The longest time to complete resolution of the IAMs was found in patients with chorea (45.7 ± 8 days); this time interval was shorter than in the patients with tremor (29.1 ± 14.9 days) ($p = 0.02$), dystonia (31.5 ± 23.5 days), and myoclonus (15 days). The severity of the disease (Table 2) was greater in patients with chorea (2 ± 0) and dystonia (1.55 ± 0.5) than in the patients with tremor (1.25 ± 0.43) and myoclonus (1 ± 0).

The Mantoux test was positive in 9 patients (64.2%); chest roentgenogram was abnormal in 5 patients (35.7%); 2 patients had pulmonary tuberculosis, which was treated one and two years earlier, respectively; Ziehl-Nielsen staining was positive in CSF in 6 patients (42.8%); the CSF culture in Jensen-Lowenstein medium was positive in 7 patients (50%); and ELISA or ADA was positive in 11 patients (78.5%). In 2 patients, the diagnosis was obtained by surgery; in one of them, the Ziehl-Nielsen and culture were positive in CSF, prior to surgery. In another patient, the diagnosis was reached by necropsy. The diagnosis of tuberculomas benefited from bacteriological confirmation in 9 patients (64.2%).

Four of the 6 patients with unilateral movement disorders had the motor deficit on the same side as the abnormal movement (Table 2). Two of the 5 patients with focal abnormal movements had ipsilateral motor deficit (Table 2). One patient with focal dystonia had tetraparesis, and another with generalized chorea had hemiparesis. The abnormal movement was ipsilateral to the hemiparesis in one of the two patients with cerebellous tuberculomas.

Table 1. Demographic characteristics, localization and diagnosis of 14 patients with intracranial tuberculomas and movements disorders

Total patients	Total number of patients (%)	Age (years)	Sex		Location of lesions			Bacteriological diagnosis	
			Male	Female	S	D	S+D	Positive	Negative
Total patients with tuberculomas	47 (100)	29.3±18.5	24	23	9	10	28	22	25
Patients with movement disorders	14 (29.7)	29.6±17.3	4	10	4	3	7	9	5
Chorea	7 (14.8)	20.2±10.9	1	6	3	2	2	4	3
Dystonia	2 (4.4)	39±3	1	1	1	-	1	1	1
Tremor	4 (8.9)	43.7±21.0	1	3	0	-	4	3	1
Myoclonus	1 (2.1)	20	1	-	0	-	1	1	-

Location of lesions: surface = S; deep = D, includes basal ganglia, thalamus, subthalamus, midbrain

Table 2. Clinical Characteristics in 14 Patients with Tuberculomas and Movement Disorders

Case No.	Age (years)	Sex	Symptom prior to admission (weeks)	Severity of disease prior to start of therapy*	Severity of disease at onset of movement disorder*	Type of movement disorder	Distribution of abnormal movement	Motor deficit	CT scan or MRI	Category of outcome*	Death
1	9	F	8	1	2	Chorea S A	Left hemi.	Left hemiparesis	Hydrocephalus, right frontal and thalamic granuloma	1	-
2	16	F	10	2	2	Chorea S, A, athetosis	Generalized	Right hemiparesis	Hyrocephalus, left thalamic granuloma	1	-
3	28	F	3	2	2	Chorea S	Right hemi.	Right hemiparesis	Hydrocephalus, left fronto-parietal and thalamic granulomas	1	-
4	22	M	8	3	2	Chorean S, A, BM	Right hemi.	Right hemiparesis	Hydrocephalus, Left caudo-putaminal-capsulo thalamic granuloma	2	-
5	8	F	10	2	2	Chorea S, A, BM	Right hemi	Right hemiparesis	Left parietal and thalamic granulomas and right cerebellous	1	-
6	17	F	4	1	2	Chorea S, A	Right upper limb	-	Granuloma and left fronto-temporal abscess	2	-
7	42	F	6 7±2.5	2	2	Chorea S, A, BM	Right upper limb	-	Right cerebellous hemispheric granuloma		+
8	31	F	8	1	1	Tremor, P, K	Right upper limb	Right hemiparesis	Right occipital and front and left front granulomas	1	-
9	25	F	6	2	2	Tremor P, K	Left upper limb	Left hemiparesis	Right parietal granuloma	1	-
10	79	M	8	1	1	Tremor P, K	Upper limbs	-	Right parietal and left front granulomas	1	-

Table 2. Clinical Characteristics in 14 Patients with Tuberculomas and Movement Disorders (cont.)

Case No.	Age (years)	Sex	Symptom prior to admission (weeks)	Severity of disease prior to start of therapy*	Severity of disease at onset of movement disorder*	Type of movement disorder	Distribution of abnormal movement	Motor deficit	CT scan or MRI	Category of outcome*	Death
11	40	F	8 7.5±0.8	2	1	Tremor P, K	Right upper limb	Left hemiparesis	Right Sylvan granuloma, hydrocephalus, right putaminal-capsulo-thalamic granuloma	1	-
12	36	M	3	2	1	Dystonia S, A, F	Left upper limb	Tetraparesis	Hydrocephalus, bilateral thalamic infarcts, bilateral Sylvan granulomas	1	-
13	42	F	4 3.5±0.5	2	2	Dystonia S, A Tremor P, K	Left upper limb	Left hemiparesis	Left cerebellar hemispheric and vermian granuloma, hydrocephalus	1	-
14	20	M	2	1	1	Myoclonus S, A	Upper and lower limbs	-	Right frontal abscess and right subdural fronto-temporal abscess	2	-

CT scan, computed tomographic scan; MRI, magnetic resonance imaging.
Plus sign indicates present, minus sign absent.
Type of chorea: spontaneous = S; intensified by action = A; with ballistic movements = BM
Type of tremor: rest = R; postural = P; kinetic = K.
Type of dystonia: spontaneous = S; intensified by action = A; mobile dystonic spasms causing repetitive dystonic posture = M; fixed present at rest and action but not intensified by action = F
Type of myoclonus: spontaneous = S; intensified by action = A; provoked by sensitive stimuli = SS
*See text for definitions

Five of the 11 patients (45.4%) (Table 2) with focal or unilateral IAMs could be correlated with a contralateral lesion. Three patients with focal or unilateral abnormal movements had isolated contralateral lesions (60%), one of them had a deep location. Two patients with focal or unilateral IAMs had more than one contralateral lesion (40%). One patient with focal dystonia and another with focal chorea had cerebellar ipsilateral isolated lesions. We found an isolated lesion in 6 (42.8%) of the 14 patients and multiple lesions in 8 (57.1%).

Chorea was generalized in 1 patient, unilateral in 4 (57.1%), and focal in 2 (28.5%) (Table 2). In 6 patients (85.7%), the chorea was intensified by action, in 3 (42.8%), it was accompanied by ballistic movements, and in 1, with athetoid postures. One patient with generalized chorea had hemiparesis. In 4 (66.6%) of the 6 patients with unilateral or focal chorea, we found hemiparesis ipsilateral to the abnormal movement.

Tremor was focal in 3 cases (Table 2). One patient with focal tremor had contralateral hemiparesis, and two had ipsilateral hemiparesis. One patient with bilateral tremor did not have any focal deficit. In all 4 patients, the tremor was postural, and in 3 of them, the tremor was kinetic. One patient with focal tremor had a focal contralateral lesion.

In two patients, dystonia was focal. In both cases, the dystonia was spontaneous and intensified by action. One patient with focal dystonia had tetraparesis and another had ipsilateral hemiparesis.

One patient with myoclonus in the four limbs had ipsilateral frontal and subdural abscesses. The myoclonus was spontaneous and intensified by action, and the patient did not show any motor deficit.

Twenty-four months after antituberculous treatment was completed, the outcome showed slight disability in 2 patients with chorea and in 1 patient with myoclonus (Table 2). One patient with chorea and AIDS syndrome died. We did not find any difference when comparing outcome in the different types of abnormal movement.

The CT or MRI, with and without contrast, of the brain showed the following abnormalities (Table 2). One patient (7.1%) had thalamic infarcts, 13 (92.8%) showed granulomas, and 1 (7.1%) had an intraparenchymatous and subdural abscess. Six patients (42.8%) had hydrocephalus. Surgery was recommended for two patients, one with chorea who had, during the antituberculous treatment, rapid and paradoxical growth of a granuloma and fronto-temporal abscess and another with myoclonus who had an intraparenchymatous lesion and another subdural. Surgery was not necessary for those patients with hydrocephalus because they were all resolved when the size of the granuloma and the edema were reduced.

Discussion

The tuberculomas are generally located in the corticomedullary junction and periventricular area [20]. They are less frequently located in the basal ganglia, brainstem, or cerebellum [3-11,20-22]. Movements disorders secondary to the presence of the tuberculomas have been infrequently reported [3-11]. In our series of patients with tuberculomas, 29.7% of them had abnormal movements.

Large series of patients with tuberculomas did not report any involuntary movements [1, 2, 21]. This could be due to the oldness of the series, which did not as yet benefit from CT scan and MRI, or some of them came from neurosurgical centers that were possibly not aware of the abnormal movements [1, 2, 21]. The difficulty of establishing an early diagnosis of tuberculomas, which in some cases is done only after surgery, the rapid improvement of the movement disorder, and the difficulty of recognizing abnormal movements and being able to differentiate them from other clinical conditions such as seizures, especially in young children, may have contributed to the paucity of reports of movements disorders [3] in some series of tuberculomas [1, 2, 21, 23, 24]. In our center, we set up standard protocols for the early identification and treatment of patients with tuberculosis of the CNS, including MRI and other methods for diagnosing tuberculosis and identifying movement disorders. In all our patients, the abnormal movements improved completely and without any treatment for the involuntary movement in a few weeks.

In our patients, a definite diagnosis of tuberculomas, including surgery and autopsy findings, was established in 64.4% of the cases, a higher proportion than in other series of patients with tuberculomas [1, 2, 21-25].

In our series, the age was different in the patients with chorea, tremor, or dystonia. The patients with tremor were the oldest. As in tuberculous meningitis [26] and other CNS infections [3], most patients with chorea were children and young people. In this study, 4 of the 7 patients with chorea were under 20 years of age, and in 6 of them chorea was unilateral or focal. A susceptibility to anatomical damage, functional reorganization of the neural circuits or probably related to cerebral plasticity could condition the appearance of a type of abnormal movement in certain age groups [27].

The severity of the disease was greater in patients who developed chorea. The patients who developed tremor had the longest interval for the post-tuberculoma presentation. The late start of a post-tuberculoma abnormal movement may result from deafferentation, due to certain functional changes in neuronal activities and their connecting structures [25].

In 50% of the cases, the abnormal movement had the same location as the focal neurological deficit. Correlation between the presence of an isolated lesion and involuntary movement was found in half of our patients.

Chorea-ballismus has been related to lesions in the subthalamic region, caudate, or putamen nucleus, globus pallidus, thalamus and cortex [3, 26, 28-30]. Thalamus nucleus lesions were the most frequent locations in our patients with chorea. In two of our patients with chorea-ballismus, we found large tuberculomas that were compromising basal ganglia and the thalamus, which could have reduced the normal excitatory drive from the subthalamic nucleus to the internal segment of the globus pallidus or inhibit output of the globus pallidus on the thalamus and give excessive excitatory drive to the cortex [28-30]. Cerebellar disorders are typically not associated with chorea phenomena, and the cerebellum or its pathways have not been usually considered in the pathophysiology of chorea [3, 26, 28-30]. In the patient with focal chorea-ballismus and whose MRI showed the presence of a cerebellar lesion ipsilateral to the chorea-ballismus syndrome, it is suggested that the abnormal involuntary movement has a cerebellar origin. This interpretation is supported by the fact that the patients, on the MRI and in the autopsy findings, do not show any other lesion.

Tremor has been associated with lesions of the basal ganglia, internal capsule, thalamus, red nucleus, rubro-olivary tract, deep cerebellar nuclei, superior cerebellar peduncle and substantia nigra, nigostriatal projection or cortex [25]. In our series, the 4 patients with tremor had supratentorial tuberculomas in the corticomedullar junction. One patient had hydrocephalus.

Usually dystonia has been attributed to the striatopallidal complex and thalamus lesions [30, 31]. In addition, rarely have focal dystonia and hemidystonia been linked to brainstem and cerebellum lesions [11, 32]. One of our 2 patients with dystonia, whose case had been published previously, had arm dystonia with an ipsilateral cerebellar tuberculoma [11], and another had thalamic infarcts and bilateral Silvian granulomas.

The intracranial tuberculomas through edema, direct pressure effect, or ischemia could compromise the excitatory or inhibitory drive of the basal ganglia or their connections with the thalamus, subthalamus or cortex [11, 27, 29]. As described in patients with stroke [33, 34], all our patients with tremor of the upper limb had cortical lesions. The high frequency of abnormal movements in patients with tuberculomas, when compared with patients with tuberculous meningitis [26], suggests that pressure mechanisms and edema in these patients contribute significantly to producing involuntary movements. This would also be supported by the relatively rapid disappearance of IAMs as a result of the antituberculous treatment. In a few cases, hydrocephalus could also be a contributing factor.

In short, movement disorders may be a frequent neurological manifestation in patients with intracranial tuberculomas. The pathogenic mechanisms responsible for movement disorders in patients with tuberculomas are multifactorial. Recognition of an involuntary movement may help to establish an early diagnosis of the tuberculomas and the therapeutic management of this treatable infection.

References

[1] Asenjo A, Valladares H, Fierra J. Tuberculomas of the brain: Report of one hundred and fifty-nine cases. *Arch Neurol Psychiatry (Chicago)* 1951;65:146-160.

[2] Dastur HM, Desai AD. A comparative study of brain tuberculomas and gliomas based upon 107 case records of each. *Brain* 1965;88:375-396.

[3] Alarcón F. Movimientos involuntarios anormales en enfermedades infecciosas. *VIII Pan-American Congress of Neurology Proceedings. October 6-12,* 1991, Montevideo, Uruguay.

[4] Alarcón F, Calderón L, Bara ME. Manejo médico de la hidrocefalia tuberculosa. *Arch de Neurobiol (Madrid)* 1985;48:133-136.

[5] Delaporte P, Salama J, Amarenco P. Tuberculome sous-thalamique révélé par un hemiballisme. *Ann Med Interne (Paris)* 1983;134:728-731.

[6] Kalita J, Ranjan P, Misra UK, Das BK. Hemichorea: a rare presentation of tuberculoma. *J Neurol Sci* 2003;208:109-111.

[7] Hoheisel G, Chan KM, Dai LK, Chan KS, Sun AJ, Luk WK, Chan CH. Involvement of the central nervous system in disseminated tuberculosis. *Dtsch Med Wochenschr* 1991;116:1228-1233.

[8] al Deeb SM, Sharif H, al Moutaery K, Biary N. Intractable hiccup induced by brainstem lesion. *J Neurol Sci* 1991;103:144-150.

[9] Kumar N, Sanchetee PC, Singh KK. Clinical and etiological profile of ataxic hemiparesis. *J Assoc Physicians India* 1996;44:383-384.

[10] Winkel M, Pagand MA, Allievi A, Kartin D, Lera G. Distonia focal y temblor secundarios a tuberculoma del tronco encefálico. *Neurología* 1998;13:250-253.

[11] Alarcón F, Tolosa E, Muñoz E. Focal limb dystonia in a patient with a cerebellar mass. *Arch Neurol* 2001;58:1125-1127.

[12] Alarcón F, Escalante L, Pérez Y, Banda H, Chacón G, Dueñas G. Tuberculous meningitis: short course of chemotherapy. *Arch Neurol* 1990;47:1313-1317.

[13] Sheller JR, Des Prez RM. CNS tuberculosis. *Neurol Clin* 1986;4:143-158.

[14] Osontokun BD, Adeuja AOG, Fumilusi JB. Tuberculous meningitis in Nigerians: a study of 194 patients. *Tropical and Geographical Medicine* 1971;25:225-231.

[15] Kurlan R, Shoulson I. Differential diagnosis of facial chorea. In Jankovic J, Tolosa E, eds. *Advances in Neurolog.* Vol. 49, Facial Dyskinesias. New York: Raven Press, 1988.

[16] Fahn S. Concept and classification of dystonia. In: Fahn S, Marsden CD, Calne DB, eds. *Advances in Neurology.* Vol. 50, Dystonia 2. New York: Raven Press, 1988.

[17] Findley LJ. *Tremors: differential diagnosis and pharmacology.* In: Jankovic J, Tolosa E, eds. Parkinson's disease and movement disorders. Baltimore, Munich: Urban & Schwarzenberg, 1988.

[18] Marsden CD, Hallet M, Fahn S. The nosology and pathophysiology of myoclonus. In: Marsden CD, Fahn S, eds. *Movement Disorders*. London: Butterworth, 1982.

[19] Obeso JA, Artieda J, Marsden CD. Different clinical presentations of myoclonus. In: Jankovic J, Tolosa E, eds. *Parkinson's Disease and Movement Disorders*. Baltimore, Munich: Urban & Schwarzenberg, 1988.

[20] Draouat S, Abdenabi B, Ghanen M, Bourget P. Computed tomography of cerebral tuberculomas. *J Comput Assist Tomogr* 1987;11:594-597.

[21] Sibley WA, O'Brien JL. Intracranial tuberculomas: a review of clinical features and treatment. *Neurology* 1956;6:157-165.

[22] Talamas O, Del Brutto OH, García Ramón G. Brain stem tuberculoma. An analysis of 11 patients. *Arch Neurol* 1989;46:529-535.

[23] van Dyk A. CT of intracranial tuberculomas with specific reference to the target sign. Neuroradiology 1988;30:329-336.

[24] Harder E, Al-Kawi MZ, Carney P. Intracranial tuberculoma: Conservative management. *Am J Med* 1983;74:570-576.

[25] Miwa H, Hatori K, Kondo T, Imai H, Mizumo Y. Thalamic tremor: case reports and implications of the tremor-generating mechanism. *Neurology* 1996;46:75-59.

[26] Alarcón F, Dueñas G, Cevallos N, Lees AJ. Movement disorders in 30 patients with tuberculous meningitis. 2000;15:561-569.

[27] Johansson BB. Brain plasticity and stroke rehabilitation. The Willis Lecture. *Stroke* 2000;31:223-230.

[28] Dewey RB, Jankovic J. Hemiballism-hemichorea: clinical and pharmacologic findings in 21 patients. *Arch Neurol* 1989;46:862-867.

[29] Dierssen G, Gioino G. Correlación anatómica de hemibalismo (sobre 116 casos publicados en la literatura). *Rev Clin Esp* 1961;82:280-305.

[30] Bhatia KP, Marsden CD. The behavioural and motor consequences of focal lesions of the basal ganglia in man. *Brain* 1994;117:859-876.

[31] Obeso JA, Giménez-Roldán S. Clinicopathological correlation in symptomatic dystonia. *Adv Neurol* 1998;50:113-122.

[32] Muñoz JE, Tolosa E, Saiz A, Vila N, Mari MJ, Blesa R. Upper limb dystonia secondary to a mid-brain hemorrhage. *Mov Disord* 1996;11:96-99.

[33] Alarcón F, Zijlmans JCM, Dueñas G, Cevallos N. Post-stroke movement disorders: report of 56 patients. *J Neurol Neurosurg Psychiatry* 2004;75:1568-1574.

[34] Kim JS. Writing tremor after discrete cortical infarction. *Stroke* 1994;25:2280-2282.

INDEX

B

C

D

E

I

J

K

L

M

N

O

P

U

V

W

Y